LEARNING FROM COVID-19

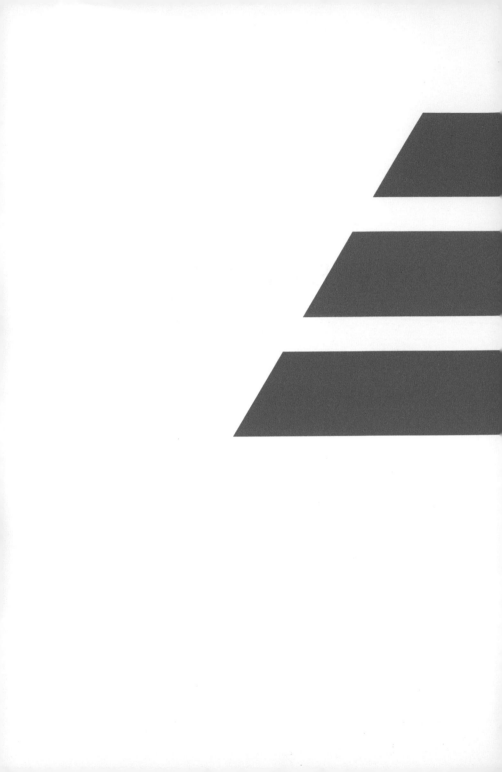

APPLYING GIS

LEARNING

FROM

COVID-19

GIS FOR PANDEMICS

Edited by
Este Geraghty, MD
Matt Artz

Esri Press
REDLANDS | CALIFORNIA

CONTENTS

PART 5: RECOVERY AND RESILIENCE 121

COVID-19: OUR LESSONS LEARNED 155

NEXT STEPS 161

INTRODUCTION

G LOBALLY, THE COVID-19 PANDEMIC BROUGHT RENEWED appreciation for the role that public health preparedness plays in keeping our communities safe. The hard lessons of the ongoing pandemic helped citizens better understand how the health of a community impacts all aspects of society. Beyond its tragic human toll, the pandemic has affected everything from the economy, transportation, and education to community design, infrastructure, and technology. Disparities in mortality rates and access to health care also emerged on the basis of race, ethnicity, and income. The scope and complexity of the crisis demonstrated that public health preparedness is a vital function. It requires careful planning and coordination across health organizations and beyond these to other members of our world ecosystem.

The global health community is in a state of reflection. As it steps back to examine the worldwide response to the pandemic, the health community can't help but be motivated to revisit health preparedness strategies and plans. *Learning from COVID-19: GIS for Pandemics* reviews the emerging lessons from the pandemic, including ways to improve our preparedness for the next health crisis.

The global response to COVID-19, the disease caused by the SARS-CoV-2 virus, highlighted the need for health organizations to engage with a wider range of collaborators. It has elevated the value of situational dashboards for communicating health issues and supporting decision-making. The pandemic magnified the importance of having the right datasets and applications to support business continuity and the recovery of our communities. Looking forward from these lessons, we value the need for equity as we build resilience at individual, organizational, and societal levels.

Organizations that prepare for and respond to public health emergencies should formally and intentionally exploit every incident as a learning experience. Many already do. Each event presents unique challenges and requires specific responses; they don't occur in isolation. These events tend to follow repeatable patterns that organizations can anticipate and employ to create healthier communities.

We have a transformational opportunity, given the magnitude of this crisis and common challenges, to build on lessons learned in response to previous public health emergencies, such as the severe acute respiratory syndrome (SARS) outbreak from 2002 to 2004, the Ebola outbreak in West Africa from 2014 to 2016, and the Zika virus epidemic from 2015 to 2016. These past emergencies produced foundational datasets, tools, models, and information products to use and share. Instead of starting from scratch, the health community can adapt and advance existing plans in the context of COVID-19 for a new crisis.

A geographic information system (GIS) is often the foundation of these efforts, turning data into location intelligence that provides agencies and civic leaders with valuable insights. More than simply mapping phenomena, GIS uses geography to furnish context for events in a common reference system. Applying spatial analysis tools, GIS brings out relationships, patterns, and associations that are often hidden by the breadth and complexity of managing multiple data inputs. What makes GIS so critical is that it supports evidence-based decision-making.

This book highlights best practices, key GIS capabilities, and lessons learned during the COVID-19 response that can help health care organizations, responders, public health programs, educators, and communities prepare for the next crisis.

Lessons from other crises

Humans are a resilient and adaptive species. Faced with armed conflicts, humanitarian tragedies, natural disasters, and health emergencies, we learn to look at situations in new ways and respond with innovation. The health community experienced this during the COVID-19 pandemic, which forced health professionals worldwide to review, rethink, and reimagine their health preparedness workflows. That spirit of invention often aligns closely with advances in technologies.

Case in point: any disease transferred to humans from other species, such as mosquito-borne malaria or West Nile virus, is a recurring worldwide threat. Early response efforts to these diseases incorporated hand-drawn maps to plan pesticide applications and paper- and PDF-based maps to visualize cases of human disease. But the past decade has seen a dramatic shift in response methods.

The 2015–2016 **Zika epidemic** brought a transition to fully integrated workflows that include surveillance, managing public requests, planning pesticide applications, and using interactive maps for public outreach and communication. Fully digital and interoperable systems helped to streamline data collection, process management, and accountability.

The lessons we're learning from applying GIS to the pandemic have implications for the way we address other human crises, even beyond the scope of this book. The ongoing **opioid epidemic**, for example, has driven innovation to address the vast range of organizational stakeholders, including not only physicians, pharmacists, and other public health professionals but also social services, public safety agencies, coroners and medical examiners, policymakers, and educators. Solutions have required a cross-sectoral and collaborative approach.

Collaborators in impacted communities have used GIS to share key data points and align jurisdictional activities around local initiatives. They also found ways to destigmatize opioid addiction in the public eye and connect residents with relevant information. For example, we saw broad participation in crowdsourcing stories of people lost to opioid overdoses as told by their loved ones. This was a new way to awaken people to the enormous toll of opioid addiction. Stories draw people in and promote empathy in ways that data, statistics, and charts never will.

Similarly, in the conversation around **homelessness**, several jurisdictions have declared states of emergency in response to this evolving crisis. That declaration is a useful political and administrative tool to raise public awareness, reallocate resources, and remove barriers to action. GIS has played an instrumental role in supporting the organizations breaking down those barriers. Communities rely on GIS to automate the collection and reporting of needed data, speed analysis and funding for mitigation efforts, and aid in the development of evidence- and consensus-based policies.

GIS has a long history when it comes to **infectious disease outbreak** response, from the plague, yellow fever, and cholera to polio, Ebola, and COVID-19. Addressing local outbreaks and a full-scale pandemic required a new paradigm of spatial thinking to facilitate decision-making, response, and recovery actions. For the first time, the health community used map-based dashboards at local and global scales to address a pandemic in near real time. The innovative use of GIS supported many strategies and programs in response to COVID-19:

- Organizations used human mobility data to estimate adherence to social distancing guidelines.

- Communities monitored the capacity of their health care systems through spatially enabled surge tools.

- Governments used location-allocation methods to distribute new resources such as testing sites and augmented care sites to locations that account for at-risk and vulnerable populations.

- Communities made information available to their residents with easy-to-use resource locators.

- Communities used maps and spatial analysis to review local case trends for guidance on easing restrictions and reopening their economies.

- Organizations used spatial thinking as they considered "back-to-workplace" plans that accounted for physical distancing and employee safety needs.

Innovation happens every day in the field of health, but now it's happening at lightning speed. Agencies must raise the standard for preparedness, response, and recovery plans because the next global crisis is just around the corner or has already arrived. For example, the outbreak of war in Ukraine in early 2022 caused a humanitarian and political crisis that threatened to engulf the world. Crises like this one, which has displaced millions of people, destroyed cities, and harmed the environment—all in the midst of a pandemic—are often interrelated and complex. GIS may be the best framework for unraveling that complexity and holistically developing the understanding that precedes informed actions and a sustained global response.

Five steps to the response

As the COVID-19 pandemic spread around the world, we became familiar with stories of social isolation and health care professionals on the front lines. A less-often told story involves the legions of

GIS professionals helping to coordinate response efforts. These people worked day and night to map the pandemic and its many ramifications, informing decision-makers and communicating to a global audience about the extent and progression of the pandemic.

This worldwide community of GIS specialists tackled innumerable challenges, the resolution of which were vital to understanding the nature and course of the disease, preparing for its arrival in new locales, and responding to its presence in our communities.

A common pattern emerged in the methods they used to respond to the crisis. It can be represented as five steps to mapping the COVID-19 pandemic.

1. **Map the cases.** Across the globe, people mapped confirmed and active cases, deaths, and recoveries to identify where COVID-19 infections existed and had occurred.

2. **Map the spread.** Time-enabled maps revealed how infections spread over time and space and where organizations should target interventions.

3. **Map vulnerable populations.** COVID-19 disproportionately affects certain population groups such as the elderly and those with underlying health conditions. Mapping social vulnerability, race, age, income, and other factors helped responders identify, monitor, and better serve at-risk groups and regions.

4. **Map capacity.** Understanding and responding to current and potential impacts of COVID-19 required awareness of the availability of medical facilities, resources, equipment, goods, and services.

5. **Communicate with maps.** Interactive web maps, dashboard apps, stories created using ArcGIS® StoryMaps℠ software, and hub sites were used to rapidly communicate an ever-evolving situation so everyone remained aware and could respond, personally and collectively, as the threat changed.

Learning from COVID-19 presents a collection of real-life stories and expert strategies that illustrate how organizations use GIS to address the challenges of pandemics. You'll see how the five steps to mapping the COVID-19 pandemic served users as an inspirational foundation for extending the uses of GIS. The book concludes with a section about getting started with GIS that provides ideas, approaches, tools, and actions that organizations can adopt to build location intelligence into decision-making and operational workflows. The stories and strategies aim to help readers integrate spatial reasoning into pandemic planning and response through the geographic lens of GIS. Using GIS, as these examples show, will help organizations better address emergencies and solve day-to-day challenges.

Many organizations realized the benefits of using GIS for the first time as they launched systems in response to the pandemic. If your organization does not use location intelligence, you can use this book to develop skills in decision-making, daily operations, and constituent satisfaction. Developing these skills does not require GIS expertise. Understanding and using location intelligence in your work simply adds another layer of knowledge to your expertise and experience. In this way, using the geographic approach for daily planning and operations can help solve problems in a real-world context.

HOW TO USE THIS BOOK

THE TERM *GEOGRAPHIC APPROACH* REFERS TO LOCATION-based analysis and decision-making. GIS professionals typically use it to study and analyze spatial problems. This book can guide your first steps with GIS to address issues that are important to you right now. Applying the geographic approach to decisions and operational processes can help solve common problems and create a more collaborative environment in your organization and community. You can use this book to identify where maps, spatial analysis, and GIS apps might be helpful in your work and then, as next steps, learn more about resources available to support you on your journey.

Learn about additional GIS resources for health and pandemic response by visiting the web page for this book:

go.esri.com/lfc-resources

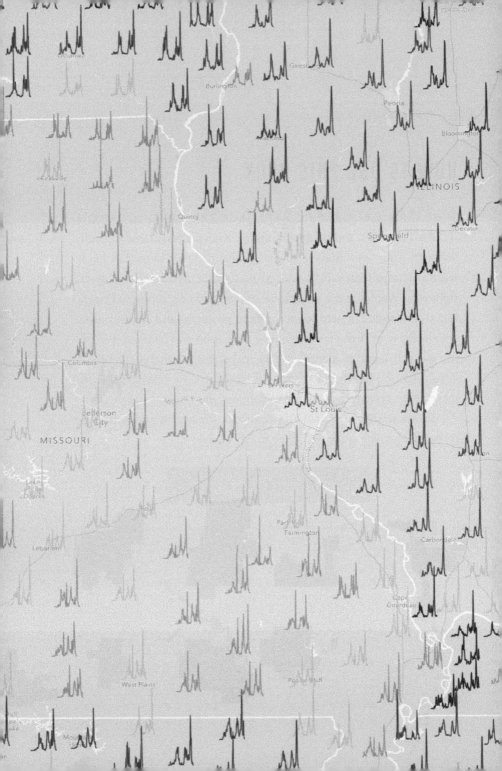

PART 1

SITUATIONAL AWARENESS

B Y DEFINITION, SITUATIONAL AWARENESS IS A SPATIAL and temporal challenge. It requires the ability to comprehend the current status of a situation and project its future status. Only when those criteria are met can leaders confidently make serious decisions about strategies, actions, interventions, and policies.

The pandemic required a level of situational awareness perhaps never before seen in a health emergency. In its sheer breadth and urgency, the pandemic brought about information needs as great as, if not greater than, any world crisis to date, including climate change, terrorism, armed conflict, displacement, and food insecurity. The unique circumstances of the pandemic required innovation around situational awareness on an unprecedented scale.

GIS quickly emerged as a key tool for managing data, visualizing information, and making informed decisions. Map-based dashboards became iconic representations of situational awareness as they tracked the pandemic at every level, but dashboards are neither simple nor the only GIS tool for creating knowledge in an emergency.

The stories in part 1 will take you on a journey beginning in early 2020 with the Johns Hopkins University (JHU) COVID-19 dashboard that opened the world's eyes to the growing outbreak in Wuhan, China. You'll learn about the practicalities of data collection, the cartographic decisions that contributed to the ominous message of the dashboard, and the architecture and automation considerations as the application (and the infection) went viral. Each decision was vital, including the one to make all underlying data open and available to the world.

The shared data from JHU enabled thousands of governments, health organizations, and businesses to consume the information, add their own local context, and inform their decision-making needs throughout the pandemic. This individualized approach was useful but insufficient. Collaboration among entities making up a state, region, or country became crucial to a coordinated response and required some level of standardization. You'll learn how the US Centers for Disease Control and Prevention (CDC) embraced map-based dashboards as a standard for communicating disease status and trends. The CDC advocated for best practices in reporting case counts, case rates, two-week trends, deaths, hospitalizations, and testing progress. And it supported the inclusion of demographic indicators such as age, gender, race, and ethnicity—showing early insight about the need to monitor for disparate impacts of the pandemic across various population groups.

The CDC project expanded on situational awareness in a way that could reasonably be called surveillance by making it possible to collect state-level dashboard data across the country for analysis and interpretation on a national scale. This effort might be considered a microcosm of the challenge of national and global disease surveillance with its multiple data inputs, required consistency in data elements, and interoperable technology components. In the big picture, public health surveillance constantly captures many kinds of data to derive true situational awareness and initiate subsequent action. One of the promising new programs is wastewater surveillance.

Testing sewage is a method that has been used before for early detection of diseases like polio. It's also been used to monitor levels of opioid drugs and their metabolites in communities and watch for dangerous spikes above baseline. More recently, wastewater surveillance programs have appeared with increasing frequency to detect SARS-CoV-2 and better understand the extent of infections in communities. For example, the University of California San Diego showed the value of geographically targeted wastewater surveillance across its campus. GIS supported the entire automated workflow, allowing real-time updates and immediate intervention. The university's integrated system of viral detection in wastewater, testing, and tracing supported a "Return to Learn" program that provided safe campus housing and allowed students to attend classes in person and conduct research.

Disease surveillance and situational awareness work in tandem as precursors to many other activities in response to the pandemic. One of those activities is contact tracing, which identifies the locations of cases and direction of spread to inform the resource needs for an appropriately scaled contact tracing effort. Through a combination of field mobility tools and dashboards, GIS has been applied to the entire process of case and contact interviews. In part 1, you'll learn how four jurisdictions in Pennsylvania (Allentown, Bethlehem, York, and Wilkes-Barre) received data from their state National Electronic Disease Surveillance System (NEDSS) and created a clear and modern process for managing contact tracing with improved efficiency and accuracy. You'll also learn how to extend traditional contact tracing for an interconnected world.

Nowadays, many of us live lives on the go. We travel by plane, train, automobile, and ship. In doing so, we interact with many strangers in the course of a day—the barista, grocery checker, or fan beside us at a sporting event. The mode and frequency of such travel stimulates community spread of disease—a stage in the pandemic in which a person may not know where or by whom they became infected. Traditional contact tracing methods are inadequate in this circumstance. Part 1 aims to expand your thinking about the importance of location information as it relates to contact tracing with the introduction of "community contact tracing." Collecting location information intentionally and strategically during a contact tracing interview can provide new insights about high-risk places and encourage new kinds of analytics that offer the opportunity to improve community safety.

Map-based situational awareness, as demonstrated by the JHU dashboard, is an effective starting point for pandemic response. Spatial and temporal information helps answer key questions about what we should do next and where.

GLOBAL DASHBOARD KEEPS TABS ON THE VIRUS

Johns Hopkins University

L ESS THAN A MONTH INTO 2020, ENSHENG DONG HEARD the news. A new viral contagion had begun to spread in Wuhan, the capital of China's Hubei province. Dong, a graduate student at Johns Hopkins University in Baltimore, was thousands of miles away from the outbreak's epicenter, but he had studied epidemics and knew how fast they can spread.

Taiyuan, another provincial capital and Dong's hometown, is about 600 miles from Wuhan. That's not exactly next door—it's the same distance that separates New York City and Detroit—but Dong felt concerned for his family's safety.

On January 20, 2020, the first US case of COVID-19 was detected in the state of Washington. For Dong, the coronavirus suddenly seemed much closer.

The next day, Dong met with his faculty adviser, Dr. Lauren Gardner, codirector of the school's Center for Systems Science and Engineering. They discussed the emerging epidemic and decided it was worth a closer look.

Gardner suggested that Dong use GIS to construct an online dashboard, a visualization tool that uses maps and data to monitor unfolding events.

Dong nodded in agreement. "That's my plan."

Civilization engineering

Dong studies systems engineering, a modernized approach to civil engineering for the complex, interconnected world.

"The emphasis is on civilization engineering," Dong said. "It's basically about the interaction of people with the built environment." The discipline allows Dong to explore ways to combine the objectivity of numeric data with the subjectivity of data visualization.

After completing his undergraduate work in China, Dong earned a master's degree in geography and statistics at the University of Idaho. While interning at the Idaho Department of Health and Welfare, he helped the agency use GIS to collect health-related data.

When Dong first contacted Gardner about the possibility of pursuing a PhD at Johns Hopkins, she was particularly intrigued by his facility with GIS, a skill Dong had honed during an internship at Esri®. He arrived on the Johns Hopkins campus a few months before his program was to start to assist in a study Gardner was coauthoring on measles vulnerability in the United States.

"I immediately jumped into the project and helped her visualize measles risk in a dashboard," he said. Media outlets, including the *New York Times* and CNN, featured Dong's handiwork, a prelude to work that would focus on a much larger health crisis on the horizon.

The data problem

GIS dashboards are typically oriented around a map, with accompanying charts, graphs, or other visuals to contextualize map imagery. But first, a dashboard requires data.

Soon after his meeting with Gardner, Dong gathered the data he needed to launch the Johns Hopkins COVID-19 Dashboard on January 21, 2020. He continued working, mostly by himself, to update data and refine the visualization, driven by a desire to map the outbreak in Taiyuan. "I wanted to see how large the dot was in my hometown and compare it to the dot in the epicenter of the outbreak," he said.

"Ensheng and I were basically the two that started the dashboard, but he was really the mastermind behind it," Gardner said in a podcast about the science behind the now-famous dashboard. "He's a total whiz with Esri technology and dashboard development."

As cases multiplied around the world, Dong struggled to keep up. He scoured the internet for reliable data, often consulting *BNO News*, a Dutch website publishing COVID-19 data from several nations in table form. In addition to gathering data, Dong had to synchronize it, accounting for the different ways governments classified cases as "confirmed" or "recovering."

Twice a day, he would update the dashboard. "For a month, I barely slept—five hours a day or less," he said.

One reason the work was so labor intensive was that Dong was inputting all the data manually. In February 2020, the ArcGIS Living Atlas of the World team at Esri helped the JHU team with "data scraping," automating the process of importing the data from China. A team of volunteers was assembled from Johns Hopkins to help update and maintain the site.

What size the dot?

Soon after Dong began to amass data, he had to confront the questions about how to present it. To emphasize the alarming nature of the pandemic, Dong chose to display bright-red dots over a stark black background. The larger the dot, the greater the number of COVID-19 cases in that region.

Behind each red dot lurks a plethora of choices. A major decision involved how to break down the data for presentation.

As Dong's team adapted the map to provide worldwide data by state and province—and, in some countries, such as the United States, by county—these choices multiplied. The county-level perspective showed the United States blanketed in red dots while other countries might have one large red dot and a lot of blank space.

At the state level for larger countries, Dong broke up one large

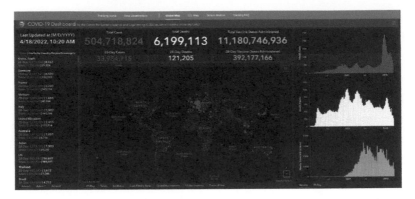

The JHU COVID-19 Dashboard has evolved over time, adding more detail to track the spread and toll of the virus.

dot so viewers could see more dots distributed in smaller sizes on the map. "That's a tricky thing for geographers," Dong said. "What's the best size for the dot?"

This kind of map must inform and empower people to act, but it also risks making people lose hope so they see no way out of the crisis.

"We're constantly adjusting the dot," Dong said. "We added a few other maps besides the cumulative and confirmed cases, such as active cases, to clearly communicate the data we were collecting and sharing. If more people in your country are recovering, you refer to that map—the dots are smaller and you feel better."

Directing increasing traffic

Increases in dashboard visitor traffic indicated broad interest in monitoring the disease's progress. "We had at least three crashes," he said. "Each time, it was because of a surge of cases in new locations. I remember that at the end of February [2020], as Italy and other European countries had more cases, we could see that a lot of Italians were jumping on the site to see what was going on."

By mid-March 2020, about the time the World Health Organization officially classified COVID-19 as a pandemic, Dong's team automated updates from all US counties.

What began as an attempt to monitor the outbreak in China has since evolved into one of the world's most trusted sources of information on the pandemic.

By the summer of 2020, the dashboard was receiving between 3 billion and 4.5 billion requests a day. "And they're coming from everywhere," Gardner said. "Most of it is just individuals clicking around on the dashboard, but there are definitely lots of requests for the data that we make available, which other groups are pulling directly into their own internal dashboards and using for policy making."

With the data gathering mostly automated, Dong could spend less time on the site and begin to study the epidemic as the basis for his doctoral dissertation. But he still keeps an eye on the map.

A version of this story by Greg Milner originally appeared as "COVID-19: Inside Look at the Johns Hopkins Dashboard, Keeping Tabs on the Virus" on the *Esri Blog* on July 16, 2020.

SUPPORTING STATE DASHBOARDS TO BETTER MONITOR CASES AND CAPACITY

US Centers for Disease Control and Prevention

EARLY IN THE PANDEMIC, THE US CENTERS FOR DISEASE Control and Prevention, or CDC, began a new effort to assist states in creating or enhancing localized COVID-19 dashboards and maps for the public.

"There's a real demand for dynamic visualizations of all kinds of data in all of our emergency responses, and particularly in this one that's affecting every US community but in a way that differs across the country," said Debra Lubar, deputy director for management and operations for the National Center for Emerging and Zoonotic Infectious Diseases at CDC.

The path of public health data goes from local to state to national levels, with state authorities aggregating details from their local colleagues. With high demand for local information about the pandemic's spread, the CDC focuses on helping states communicate this data to the public. Dashboards displaying data and maps to convey COVID-19 case locations and counts have become the standard for communicating status and trends in the global pandemic.

"There are critical data elements that are really important for people to see about their communities, where their families live, or places they plan to travel," Lubar said.

Presenting health data to the public

In normal circumstances, the CDC partners closely with state public health agencies and issues grant awards to assist with internal data collection and disease surveillance. During the pandemic, the CDC has focused more externally on helping states deliver data to residents, civic leaders, and public health administrators.

"We've seen that many states, including New York, South Dakota, and South Carolina, have been communicating effectively with the public, providing substantial granularity and transparency," Lubar said. "CDC will continue providing support that will help states improve these efforts. We've worked to ease their participation, in part by recognizing that different states may have different needs."

The arrival of a new disease brought innovative efforts to deliver cutting-edge technology to state public health professionals so they could display their own data. "CDC is providing access to tools and funding to state health departments that are leading public health actions in response to the pandemic," Lubar said.

While the work isn't focused on standards or mandates, the CDC has shared best practices and guidance based on the kinds of questions it has fielded. The basic data points include case counts, case rates, and recent trends for cases, deaths, hospitalizations, and testing. "We've also encouraged states to add relevant demographic data, such as racial, ethnic, gender, and age information," Lubar said.

With this information, states and localities can better monitor impacts and mitigate risks, and federal resources can go where they are needed most, because all parties are working from the same data.

Unprecedented in so many ways

Counting and reporting details about each person infected with COVID-19 presents new challenges for public health officials. Apart from exceptions such as foodborne illnesses and influenza, most infectious diseases in the modern era have low case numbers, and outbreaks have been rare events with limited scope.

An outbreak involving the food supply can impact thousands of people, and each case is counted. Most outbreaks are quickly investigated and halted. Influenza, on the other hand, impacts millions of people annually, and a combination of surveillance and scientific methods can be used to reliably estimate the impact and outcomes instead of counting each case.

"The way we're tracking this disease [COVID-19] is really different," Lubar said. "Our systems have to grow and flex to accommodate a pandemic where it's important to know about each case and be able to trace the contacts."

Better information about the location of cases has taken on greater importance.

"Understanding where cases are occurring is critical to understanding how disease is spreading," Lubar said. "New technology, combined with the globalization of the world population and trade, has really shown us new ways that diseases spread. Spatial analysis is critical to that."

CDC also uses mapping to monitor the spread of disease at the county level and reaches out to states to help if it detects a spike in the number of cases.

Dashboards help states remain vigilant

CDC contracted with Esri, an international supplier of GIS services and products, including ArcGIS Dashboards, to build or enhance publicly available COVID-19 data dashboards. (Editor's note: Mention of Esri and its products and services does not constitute an endorsement by CDC.) The effort focused on the need to provide easily accessible and transparent information to guide mitigation measures.

At first, several states didn't have a dashboard. Through this contract, they could request tools and services to build one. States that had dashboards could request enhancements, such as automating data workflows, exposing services or the application programming interface (API), to improve sharing and collaboration, and applying best practices to data flows and visualizations. Each CDC and Esri engagement with a state lasted between one and three weeks.

The work on dashboards was part of a larger data modernization and transparency initiative at the CDC. The dashboard project provided one way to improve consistent and reliable information to monitor COVID-19 cases across the country, giving states and CDC the insight they needed to act.

"We wanted to be ready, and the data helped us," Lubar said.

The enhanced reporting effort also helped states and CDC learn more about the pandemic to continually improve surveillance systems and approaches to protect public health, she added.

"We'll continue to learn from the arc of this outbreak for years to come," Lubar said.

A version of this story by Este Geraghty originally appeared as "COVID-19: CDC Supports State Dashboards to Better Monitor Cases and Capacity" on the *Esri Blog* on July 9, 2020.

IT'S IN THE WASTEWATER: SENSING AND MAPPING COVID-19

University of California San Diego

B Y MIDSUMMER 2021, THE DELTA VARIANT HAD BECOME widespread, toppling any optimism that the COVID-19 pandemic might end soon. But a team at the University of California San Diego (UCSD) had already spotted this new threat. There it was, the virus's RNA sequence, in wastewater samples.

Rather than cause alarm, the presence of the more infectious COVID-19 variant offered the team hope. Here was evidence that its epidemiological strategy could detect the Delta variant and likely any future mutations.

The UCSD program to detect and communicate COVID-19 cases involved daily wastewater testing. Results were tied to a live map, created with GIS, to show which university buildings had a positive reading. The virus sensing effort from sewage led to early viral testing recommendations for individuals, which, in turn, helped curb campus spread. This effort enabled UCSD to offer on-campus housing and in-person classes and research opportunities through most of the pandemic.

Although other campuses have attempted similar screening programs, few reached UCSD's scale or efficiency. To be successful, the system needed to provide near real-time information. As evidence of its achievement, the UCSD team was tapped to monitor wastewater for the city of San Diego's approximately 1.4 million residents using the same innovative process.

How UCSD led its Return to Learn program

The campus setting proved to be an ideal location for devising disease surveillance systems and curbing the spread of COVID-19, even though people were living and working in close quarters.

The university launched its Return to Learn program with three pillars in mind: risk mitigation, viral detection, and intervention. The university's Office of Operational Strategic Initiatives led the effort, with Rob Knight, professor and director of the Center for Microbiome Innovation, as the chief laboratory investigator.

Concerned that outbreaks could occur and spread rapidly in buildings with high occupancy, Knight and his team began testing wastewater as a way to safely maintain the campus population during the pandemic and take early action when needed.

Often, infected students were not aware they had the virus. In the summer of 2020, the system detected a positive case one Friday

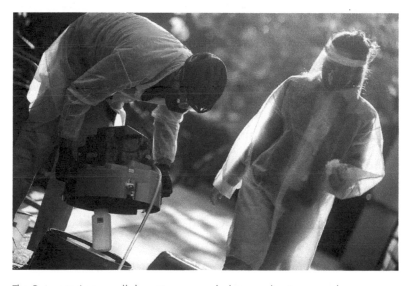

The Return to Learn collaboration expanded to academic researchers, students, and campus staff, including facilities management, planning, emergency response, health, dining and hospitality, and other departments. (Wastewater testing image courtesy of UCSD.)

afternoon. Notifications went out within 14 hours, and that weekend more than 650 people were tested. Two asymptomatic individuals tested positive and self-isolated, preventing a larger outbreak.

The Return to Learn team credited transparency as the key to participation. Detailed maps of every building, pipe, and sewage access point formed the basemap. A public GIS dashboard showed daily updates of monitored buildings, sampled water, and detected virus. The dashboard kept the entire campus community abreast of the university's viral infection status.

"It's not just our processing of the data but being able to share that data out to everyone and the public," said Natasha Martin, an associate professor in the Department of Medicine, Division of Infectious Diseases and Global Public Health at UCSD. "We have people that visit, and they can check on the public dashboard and see if a particular building was positive on that day."

Despite early uncertainty about how well the system would detect cases, it proved to be extremely sensitive, Martin said. More than 85 percent of the university's residential cases were detected in the wastewater.

Showing students and staff where the virus is

At the outset, UCSD had just six wastewater autosamplers that captured effluent for laboratory testing. The results were recorded manually in a spreadsheet. But soon the university was sampling the wastewater in 350 buildings every day, and the results were automatically added to the map.

To achieve automation, UCSD created a better map that included sewer system pathways to correlate wastewater samples collected in pipes to the buildings they served. Once a building was identified, the university traced the virus to individuals through standard nasal-swab testing.

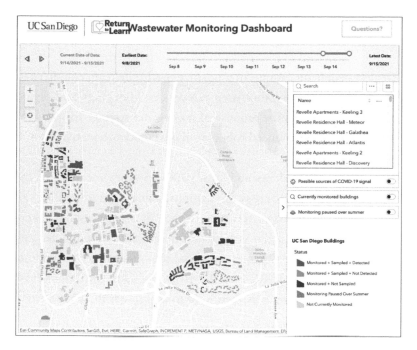

The GIS trace tool automatically pushes wastewater test results to a public map and notification repository. A suite of Esri tools, including ArcGIS Pro, ArcGIS Online, ArcGIS Notebooks, and ArcGIS Survey123, was used for different elements of the wastewater monitoring effort.

During the summer of 2020, the Return to Learn team began issuing notifications to campus residents and staff by email, lobby fliers, and even door-to-door knocking to compel further testing. To the surprise of Martin and others, it worked. When people received notifications of positive wastewater samples, individual testing rates increased as much as 13-fold. The testing prompted a quick start to isolation and contact tracing.

Automation involves robots, dashboards, maps, and listservs

To alert people on campus of a positive result, the team couldn't rely on a time-consuming multistep lab process. Backlogs and delays would have derailed the promise of wastewater testing. To speed the process, UCSD introduced robots to the lab and automated the notification systems.

A group of students and staff gathered every morning to collect sewage samples across the campus, using liquid-handling collection robots, and then returned to the lab for processing. There, robots concentrated the virus using magnetic nanoparticles and then extracted RNA—genetic material that makes up the genomes of viruses such as SARS-CoV-2—from the samples. Polymerase chain reaction testing was then used to search for the virus's signature genes.

The automated, high-throughput system could process 24 samples every 40 minutes. Data was then added to a digital dashboard and map that tracked new positive cases building by building.

If Martin already knew that a student was isolating in a building from which a positive sample returned, she didn't issue a notification. The notification process was otherwise fully automated. Martin provided the dates of positivity and the sampler number, and emails were sent automatically to everyone living or working in that building.

She estimated that automation initially saved her two to three hours per day. Without automation, it would have been hard to expand the scale of the wastewater testing effort.

Expanding beyond the campus

With the promise of curtailing future epidemics and pandemics, wastewater surveillance could be a university's or community's greatest early warning system. Recognizing the efficacy of wastewater testing, the CDC launched its National Wastewater Surveillance System in September 2020.

"We hope wastewater-based epidemiology will become more widely adopted," Knight said in March 2021. "Rapid, large-scale infectious disease early alert systems could be particularly useful for community surveillance in vulnerable populations and communities with less access to diagnostic testing and fewer opportunities to distance and isolate—during this pandemic, and the next."

A version of this story by Este Geraghty originally appeared as "It's in the Wastewater: How UC San Diego Senses and Maps COVID-19" on the *Esri Blog* on September 28, 2021.

A NEW TOOL FOR CONTACT TRACING

Esri

THE COVID-19 PANDEMIC REQUIRED US TO FACE NEW challenges and find new opportunities in our response to a global health crisis. One such opportunity, community contact tracing, offered a technology-driven update to traditional contact tracing methods.

Contact tracing begins with the understanding that a person's risk of contracting a virus relates directly to their exposure to people who are already infected. Public health professionals use contact tracing to break disease transmission chains with the goal of preventing the spread of infection. The process starts when a contact tracer interviews someone infected with a contagious or communicable disease.

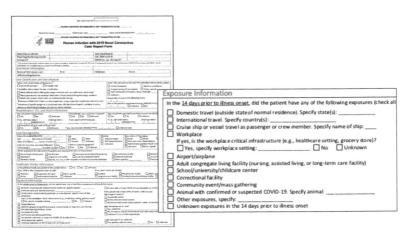

The CDC's standard form for contact tracing does not capture location data in a usable way. A small change to the exposure information section could enable valuable new analyses.

The contact tracer asks the infected person, designated as *confirmed case,* about their close contacts during a specific period. Through empathic questioning, the tracer assesses symptoms and gather details about the person's exposure. The tracer typically provides resources for testing and medical care and offers guidance on isolating safely to prevent disease transmission.

Conventional contact tracing was typically a manual process. The CDC published a standard form and methodology specifically for the COVID-19 response. Unfortunately, the established process did not systematically capture useful location information. To support the process of contact tracing, Esri introduced the concept of Community Contact Tracing in the summer of 2020.

The need for community contact tracing

In the earliest stage of an outbreak, when we observe human-to-human transmission of infection, contact tracing becomes an effective containment intervention. However, as an outbreak evolves into a pandemic, transmission advances to community spread—a situation in which infected people may not be sure how, where, or when they contracted the virus. This is where a location-focused approach can help.

The COVID-19 pandemic quickly transitioned to a community spread phase. Although contact tracing normally does not continue at this phase, public health authorities worldwide continued asking for contact tracing to be scaled to unprecedented levels in an effort to prevent further spread of the virus. To succeed in these conditions, specialists needed to think and work differently.

Esri believed that the person-to-person approach inherent in traditional contact tracing should expand to include person-to-person-to-place—a simple innovation with big returns. Adding *place* to the approach makes sense in our highly complex, highly mobile, and interconnected world.

Benefits of community contact tracing

Adding location information to contact tracing allows public health analysts to perform spatial analysis and illuminate the places where viral spread is happening outside of direct and prolonged contact between two individuals.

Tools such as link analysis and centrality can identify places that may connect disease transmission between confirmed cases and contacts otherwise unknown to one another. Spatially based link analysis identifies relationships and connections not easily seen in raw data, while centrality is a measure of importance for nodes in a network. Such tools capture the importance of person-to-person-to-place

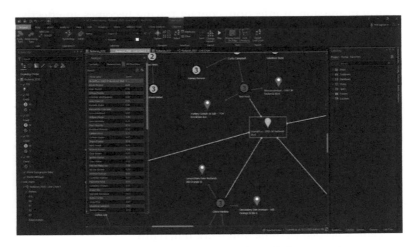

Using ArcGIS Pro, connections between people and places can be uncovered with a combination of link analysis and centrality analysis, which determines the importance of a node within the network. In this fictional dataset, Home Plus connects several cases that are unknown to each other and had no other transmission contacts in their network.

relationships. Consider the example of a confirmed case infecting a contact when they shop at the same home improvement store. When the store is identified as the place of transmission, decision-makers could opt to have the location disinfected and tighten social distancing rules.

As we confront the challenges of COVID-19, spatial technologies allow us to think differently. Public health professionals are contemplating innovative ways to scale contact tracing efforts, recognizing that community contact tracing uncovers important insights to advance interventions.

Public health departments can use GIS to perform location analytics, which involves examining collected data to quickly identify potential contacts and determine where specific cases might originate. With a location-focused supplement to traditional contact tracing, community contact tracing offers increased odds of containing COVID-19 or any other community spread contagion.

A version of this story by Este Geraghty originally appeared as "COVID-19: Introducing Community Contact Tracing" on the *Esri Blog* on June 25, 2020.

GIS-BASED CONTACT TRACING INITIATIVE SETS US PRECEDENT

Cities of Allentown, Bethlehem, York, and Wilkes-Barre, Pennsylvania

WHEN VICKY KISTLER, THEN DIRECTOR OF HEALTH FOR Allentown, Pennsylvania, and Matt Leibert, the city's chief information officer, traveled together to an Esri conference in Philadelphia in 2003, they had high hopes for what GIS could provide for their city, imagining that one day advanced technology could help them visualize and track the spread of disease in real time. Little did they know then that a global pandemic would give them the chance to adopt this capability.

Working with the cities of Bethlehem, York, and Wilkes-Barre, Allentown in 2020 took the lead on a GIS-based community contact tracing initiative that underpinned one of the United States' more promising responses to the COVID-19 pandemic.

The limitations of an app-based model

When the pandemic arrived, many local governments turned to app-based solutions for contact tracing and exposure notification as they tried to keep up with the spread of the virus. Unfortunately, cities often found themselves in situations in which app-based models failed to gain momentum, resulting in ineffective adoption rates. So state and local governments relied mostly on traditional manual processes as they determined the scale of their contact tracing workforces.

As the pandemic continued, transmission advanced to community spread, a situation in which people could not pinpoint how they got infected. Community spread makes identifying and tracking contacts much more difficult. For this reason, it's useful to adopt a location-focused approach.

For the COVID-19 pandemic, the solution was far more complicated than downloading apps and building the workforce, said Matt Leger, policy research analyst for the Innovations in Government Program at Harvard Kennedy School. Tracing programs face significant operational constraints aggravated by often outdated back-end IT infrastructure that slows responses, said Leger, who also serves as director of strategy at CONTRACE Public Health Corps, a social enterprise that provides contact tracing workforce solutions to the public and private sectors.

However, combining person-to-person tracing with upgraded IT infrastructure and GIS tools can help overcome these limitations.

Layers of benefits to using GIS

Allentown addressed the challenge of tracking viral spread by using community contact tracing tools from Esri. As Kistler and Leibert explained, the tools gave Allentown a running start because it already used ArcGIS software. The city invested in IT solutions several years ago in hopes that the investment would increase productivity.

This foresight, which included broadening the city's GIS capacity, produced benefits for both routine and extraordinary service demands. GIS tools helped Allentown replace cumbersome, paper-based processes with digital technology and semiautomated workflows. ArcGIS also served as the foundation for standardization and collaboration among the four cities participating in the community contact tracing initiative.

Joseph Yashur, community health specialist for the City of Bethlehem, agreed that successful contact tracing required new capabilities. He noted that tasks that once took hours to complete, including performing quality assurance on the data, are done much more efficiently using tools such as ArcGIS Survey123.

Myriad advantages for the community

For the four Pennsylvania cities participating in this initiative, the now automated and spatially oriented workflows that connect case investigation and contact tracing have produced substantial advantages as community contact tracing has accelerated. Examples of the many manual steps that have been automated to improve efficiency include verifying addresses and notifying contact tracing staff when there is a rapid reassignment of cases.

Since the spatial approach to contact tracing increases the ability of city leaders to inform the public and enact strategic, place-based interventions, accuracy is key.

The GIS-based contact tracing tools used in the four cities

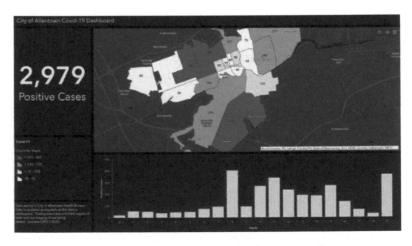

Officials from the City of Bethlehem appreciate that cities and counties in Pennsylvania are sharing data and borrowing technology ideas from one another.

reduced human errors that can occur in manual data entry and analysis. These tools protect people's privacy and provide dashboards and map narratives of COVID-19 cases to help viewers visualize what is happening. This information, in turn, can improve community safety.

Geographic analysis can also connect locations of the disease to affected individuals and nearby resources. As the pandemic continued, Allentown planned to integrate an automated notification system for high-risk neighborhoods and for residents who were exposed to someone who tested positive.

Looking ahead to future public health uses

Having a cloud-based platform allows Allentown to share innovations and discoveries with other public health departments. Kistler emphasized that collaboration and sharing ideas can enhance Allentown's capabilities even further.

The GIS-based foundation allowed many agencies to gain even broader insight into public health. Bethlehem and Allentown public health leaders hope that the layered data that GIS provides will help cities pay more attention to the social determinants of health. Officials were considering the application of GIS technology to trace sexually transmitted diseases (STDs), tuberculosis, whooping cough, and other illnesses. And the four cities in the collaborative are optimistic that, by connecting health data with geographic data, they can join together to apply for research grants and respond to the causes of health disparities.

Kristen Wenrich, Bethlehem's health director, said her city also hoped to use GIS technology for other disease prevention strategies once officials grew more familiar with the capabilities of spatial analysis.

"When you see mapped clusters, you can also see potential action that can be taken," Wenrich said.

For example, the capabilities of GIS analysis, mapping, and visualization helped Bethlehem improve outreach efforts to Spanish-speaking communities after the public health department saw the disproportionate impact of COVID-19 in certain Hispanic neighborhoods.

As an investment, the transition to GIS has continued to provide returns for an effective pandemic response and for public health and city government in general.

A version of this story by Stephen Goldsmith originally appeared as "GIS-Based Contact Tracing Initiative in Pennsylvania Sets US Precedent" in the Fall 2020 issue of *ArcNews*.

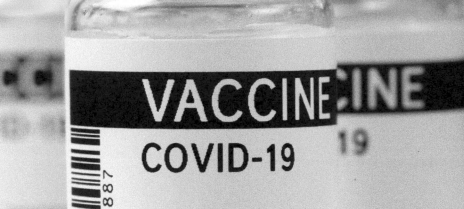

PART 2

EQUITABLE RESOURCE ALLOCATION

J UST ABOUT EVERYTHING GIS DOES TO SUPPORT HEALTH and pandemic response also relates to improving equity. When we map information, we search for patterns and relationships in our data to pinpoint disparate outcomes, gaps in service availability, and poor access to existing services. We employ spatial analytics to explain current and emerging patterns, which then informs our planning and decision-making for applying resources to achieve beneficial results. Desired impacts are well defined and measurable through map-based dashboards and communication hubs. This work is health GIS in a nutshell.

This section explores various perspectives on the concept of equity and the need to be smart and strategic about resource allocation. The challenge of applying these concepts and strategies in a pandemic is that there is no time to waste. Having situational insight, as discussed in part 1, underlies everything that comes next. Building on that foundation will help responders spot equity issues and apply mitigation strategies more quickly.

The first story in this section addresses the issue of racial inequities during COVID-19. The pandemic illustrated and magnified the deep-rooted structural racism that exists in societies around the world. Increased awareness of racism as a societal crisis is evidenced by many declarations of a public health state of emergency. We must address inequities in health care for Blacks, Latinos, and other communities of color in any pandemic response. Other vulnerable communities, including the world's poorest people, have borne a disproportionate amount of sickness and death in the pandemic. For whatever inequities we face, the lessons of this section tell us that we must ask the right questions, acquire the right data, perform meaningful analysis, and act.

Often, geography plays a crucial role in the equity issue. The ability to get tested, vaccinated, and treated depends on geographic access. Pandemic responders must figure out the best locations to deploy resources so that people can get the timely care they need. But finding access gaps is not always a straightforward process. Simply drawing a buffer of a certain distance around a place and equating that to thresholds of adequate access on a map is no longer good enough. For example, a distance of 10 miles can require vastly different travel times and travel experiences, depending on location, time of day, mode of transportation, and even the topography. GIS can calculate specific access parameters when underlying road network data is available, but that's not always the case. But even without that data, we can use globally available datasets to estimate travel times. Using spatial thinking, we can manage resource allocation to address access gaps, even in the most rural areas or least developed countries.

Among the resources most needed during the pandemic were widespread testing locations and vaccination venues. GIS supported the most common question regarding these resources: "Where shall we site them?" To develop efficient processes, pandemic responders across the globe used GIS to help manage crowds at the testing locations, maintain social distancing at those sites, and consider a rapidly expanding array of perspectives in allocating vaccine resources.

COVID-19 vaccines might be considered the most precious resource available in the battle to control the pandemic. Such a precious and limited resource—the World Health Organization noted that vaccine shortages and inequities had a disproportionate impact on low- and middle-income countries—raises many questions and considerations with a spatial component:

- Where can we set up vaccine distribution locations?

- Where can we store the vaccine, given cold-chain requirements?

- How do we redistribute vaccine?

- How can we identify and eliminate vaccine inequities?

- Where do we need to prioritize populations at increased risk?

Part 2 shows how GIS helped pandemic responders address the need for equitable vaccine distribution at local, county, state, and national levels. These real-life stories reveal common patterns and individual innovations in the use of GIS that can support the global vaccine effort going forward.

Responsible organizations and resilient community planners strive to deliver pandemic resources, such as testing and vaccine sites, in the right locations. But the concept of equitable resource allocation cannot stop there. Sometimes, resources must be delivered to people right where they live. This challenge is also a spatial problem, one that Clackamas County, Oregon, addressed when it used the routing capabilities of GIS to deliver vaccines directly to homebound residents. GIS tools helped the responders do their job twice as fast.

Because speed is paramount in a crisis, pandemic responders cannot afford to make costly, time-consuming mistakes in allocating health resources. They must also consider the differing needs of vulnerable communities. If not attended to, health disparities can deepen and outcomes worsen. GIS can help reveal and simplify complex patterns and multiple information sources to help ensure no one is left behind.

ANALYZING RACIAL INEQUITIES DURING COVID-19

Esri

COVID-19 CASE DATA REVEALS INEQUITIES AMONG RACIAL groups, largely driven by entrenched systemic inequalities. Urgent and racially equitable crisis relief requires organizations to understand the content and context of racial marginalization and its impacts. In other words, making progress begins with good data.

Accessing data for analysis

As a starting point, ArcGIS Living Atlas (livingatlas.arcgis.com) contains authoritative data layers with information about various demographic characteristics. The site includes an array of data on race, ancestry, language, income, age, education, employment, and more. Each data layer aggregates variables at state, county, and census tract geographics. These different geographic scales enable analysis of disparities and inequities at local, state, and national levels. You can use ArcGIS Online and ArcGIS Pro to incorporate these data layers into relevant maps and applications. Combining and overlaying sociodemographic data layers with organizational data can help you learn more about the needs of unserved and underserved communities in your geographic area of interest.

A starting point for racial equity analysis

A racial equity analysis begins with relevant questions. Who is most at risk and where are they located? Can systemically disadvantaged communities readily access existing resources such as health care providers, broadband, and other critical supports during the pandemic? Where can pandemic responders deploy new emergency resources (such as food distribution centers, pop-up health clinics, and testing and vaccination sites) to ensure equitable access for everyone?

Ensuring equity involves identifying vulnerable populations and assessing racial, health, and economic equity for COVID-19 mitigation based on these and other risk factors:

- Areas with higher numbers and proportions of people of color

- Percentage of residents in an area experiencing multidimensional health risks, such as food insecurity, poverty, senior population, and populations with a physical disability

- Neighborhoods with few or no bank branches (banking deserts), generally within a 10-mile radius, making it harder to cash checks, access deposits, and seek loans

- Neighborhoods lacking access to healthy, affordable food (food deserts)

- Percentage of people in an area working in industries where they are at higher risk of losing their jobs and wages.

- Percentage of homes without broadband internet access

Populations and areas identified with increasing numbers of these risk factors often have higher COVID-19 mortality rates and lack equitable access to testing, vaccines, and other health resources.

Breaking down and building up the data

An analysis of racial and other inequities involves disaggregating data by race, ethnicity, gender, language, income, and other demographic factors to the extent possible. Breaking data points down to the smallest possible geography better detects inequities and informative

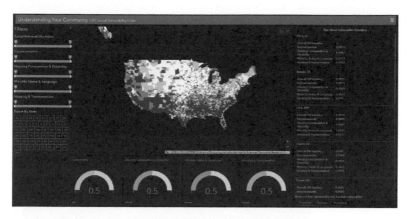

The CDC Social Vulnerability Index ranks every county and census tract in the United States by its social vulnerability.

patterns in the data. Disaggregating data at hyperlocal geographies is critical because vulnerable communities often include members with many different disadvantages; highly aggregated data may hide or mask the problem. An equitable response will devote resources in proportion to the degree of vulnerability and need.

While disaggregated data is most useful when preparing to take local action, building indices that combine variables offers a broader view. For example, the CDC's Social Vulnerability Index helps users understand the intersection of multiple risk factors. Mapping this index with key outcomes of interest and demographic characteristics such as age and race may reveal connections that deserve deeper consideration and analysis. The index may also be explored independently in an application such as the Understanding Your Community dashboard.

Analyzing for action

Spatial analysis often works best when it focuses on solving specific problems to meet a community's greatest needs. For example, to

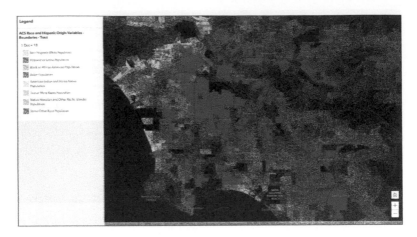

A map showing population density by race, such as this one for Los Angeles, can be compared with other data, such as income, housing, medical providers, and the locations of other resources, to address health care needs in vulnerable communities.

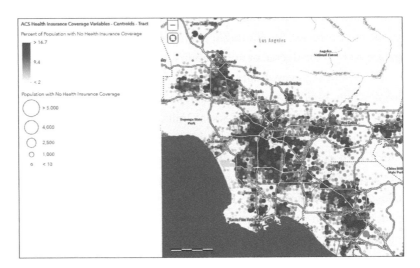

This map showing populations without health insurance in Los Angeles can be used to coordinate social safety net programs that offer financial support for health care.

determine the best location for food resources, analysts could compare data on families who do not have a car to data on children who qualify for free or lower-cost lunches in communities of color. Such a comparison might reveal the need for a food pantry or school-based site to distribute food within a reasonable walking distance from people's homes.

Spatial analysis can also identify ways to support families without health insurance. Immigrant populations, especially undocumented immigrants, often lack access to social safety net programs that offer financial support for health care and its costs.

You can identify and develop strategies to meet these needs proactively by mapping where food and health care resources exist in relation to people without health insurance.

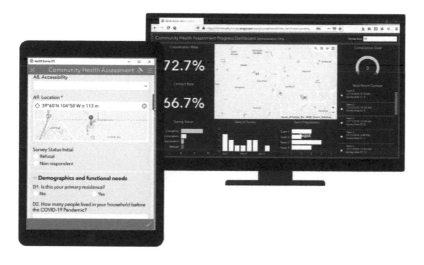

Community health assessments to determine the health care needs and challenges of residents—ranging from access to healthy foods to the availability of prescription medicines—can be conducted in the field with results viewed in real time.

Addressing data gaps

Although data is increasingly available, it's still common to encounter data gaps for specific populations of interest. In these cases, several GIS tools can help automate data collection. For example, Esri's Community Health Assessment Solution and Coronavirus Response Solution include survey templates and data collection tools that help close data gaps.

A version of this story by Clinton Johnson, Margot Bordne, and Rebecca Lehman originally appeared as "Analyze Racial Inequity during COVID-19" on the *ArcGIS Blog* on April 14, 2020.

SPATIAL APPROACHES TO DETERMINING ACCESSIBILITY

Esri

I N THE CONTEXT OF INTERNATIONAL DEVELOPMENT, accessibility is a concept often applied in understanding whether residents can reach schools, health centers, infrastructure, or jobs with reasonable effort when necessary. This is important to maximize positive outcomes and ensure more inclusive development. In the same way, accessibility is a key consideration for equitable resource allocation during a pandemic.

GIS offers multiple approaches to evaluate accessibility. The most commonly used spatial technique to evaluate accessibility is through a network analysis. In a network analysis, a key factor is an accurate network dataset, containing information about the underlying transportation network (roads, paths, trails, and so on), associated speed limits, directionality, connectivity, surface types, and more. It is used to calculate how far an individual can travel in a specified time by various modes of transport, such as walking or driving. Network analysis can also be applied to datasets such as the General Transit Feed Specification (GTFS) to determine accessibility based on public transportation schedules.

While network analysis is a proven way to evaluate accessibility, its use is limited by the availability of a network dataset. For example, in regions with the greatest need for aid, such as sub-Saharan Africa and southeast Asia, network data is available only for major highways, which has marginal use when seeking to calculate health service accessibility in rural and underserved regions. Nevertheless, it is possible to quantify accessibility, even in the absence of a network dataset, by applying spatial analysis to geographic features such as elevation, land cover, and others.

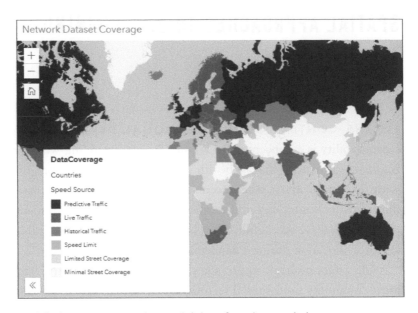

A global perspective on the availability of road network datasets:
progressively darker shades of green indicate more detailed street and
traffic information, to the point of predicting future traffic patterns.

The conceptual approach

Before learning how to determine accessibility using tools in ArcGIS
Pro at the functional level, a high-level conceptual overview of the
approach may be helpful.

In the absence of network data, the quickest way to model accessibility is by creating a buffer around a location. For example, to
generate a buffer to estimate the distance a person can walk in 30
minutes from their home, you can create a buffer with a radius of
2.5 kilometers, assuming an average walking speed of 5 kilometers
per hour. While this may be a fair approximation in urban settings
where walking time may be predictable, there are obvious limitations
in rural areas. The walking pace may vary depending on the slope of
the terrain (flat versus steep), the type of surface (pavement versus

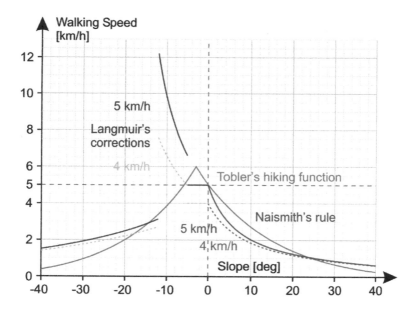

Various models of walking speed versus slope. Note that Tobler's hiking function (the green line) peaks at −3 degrees.

mud), and the presence of geographic barriers such as rivers, lakes, and mountain ranges.

To overcome these limitations, accessibility can be modeled using topography, which, in part, is represented by raster layers such as digital elevation models (DEM). In this approach, a DEM is used to calculate the slope of the terrain, and the slope is used to determine the maximum walkable speed. Using models like Tobler's hiking function associates maximum walking speeds with slope (see in the graph where 6 kilometers per hour of walking speed is achieved when the downward slope is −3 degrees). Modeling walking speed is not limited to Tobler's hiking function as there are other models (for example, Naismith's rule) that may be used to predict walking speed based on slope.

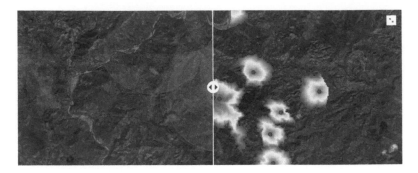

A comparison of accessibility using the buffer method (left) versus the geographic features approach (right).

To further refine the model and improve accuracy, analysts can introduce barriers and costs. For example, one can assume that individuals will not swim across rivers, even though crossing a river may represent the shortest physical distance from their location to their destination. In this context, geographic features of rivers can be modeled as impassable barriers. That same logic can be applied to other geographic features, such as mountains, dense forests, and lakes.

In addition to introducing barriers to the model, it is also possible to incorporate impedances. These are circumstances that hinder progress along the network to be traveled. For example, paved roads are easier to walk than dirt trails, and dirt trails are easier to walk than agricultural or wooded land. In network analysis these variances in walkable surface types can be modeled through cost surfaces, which introduce impedances, or costs, to walking across an area given the nature of its walkable surface. Let's consider a publicly available land cover dataset from ArcGIS Living Atlas along with free and editable road data from OpenStreetMap. Three surface types—roads, grassland, and forests—can be derived from the data, representing low to high impedance, respectively. Then each surface can be given a numeric score (1–3) to model their relative difficulty,

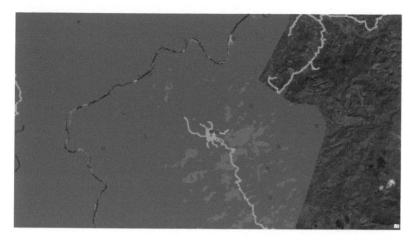

An example cost surface overlaid on a satellite image shows three categories: urban and road (green), areas of minimal vegetation (purple), and forests (orange).

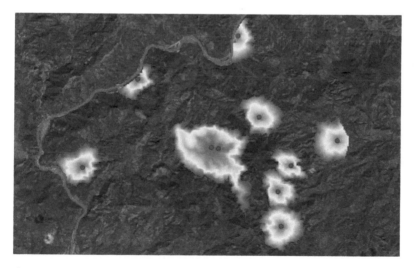

The output polygon from the model represents the outer boundary in which an individual can walk from a starting point (red dots) to a location within one hour (orange outer border of polygons).

1 being the easiest to walk on and thus the quickest. A surface type with a value of 2 is considered twice as difficult to walk as a surface type with a value of 1, and so on.

Travel times and distances can be approximated in the absence of a network dataset by incorporating a DEM, rivers, land cover, and road data layers.

For more detail on the technical approach followed in this story, see the link to "Spatial approaches to determining accessibility" at go.esri.com/lfc-resources.

Conclusion

Even in places where data is missing or incomplete, the geographic approach allows us to address issues of access to care, services, and equitable resource allocation in a data-driven way. We can use this approach anywhere.

A version of this story by Calvin Kwon and Liz Graham originally appeared as "Spatial Approaches to Determine Accessibility" on the *ArcGIS Blog* on April 1, 2021, and was updated on June 9, 2021. The graph on page 43 is courtesy of Wikipedia.

GIS HELPS ACHIEVE EQUITABLE, SPEEDY VACCINE DISTRIBUTION

Esri

A S FINAL APPROVALS FOR A COVID-19 VACCINE WERE ON track and distribution of the vaccine was expected in late 2020, governments worldwide prepared to distribute vaccines on a massive scale—an effort that included the hurdles of meeting subzero storage requirements, prioritizing vulnerable communities, communicating with each other and the public, and ensuring equity across geographies large and small.

The work to safely develop and plan immunizations in the United States and worldwide required the most complex global vaccination campaign in history. From the pandemic's onset, government and health care leaders relied on ArcGIS technology for real time visualization dashboards, data sharing, analysis, and planning. The same GIS approach proved crucial for vaccine distribution.

Leaders needed to fine-tune vaccination scenarios related to priority and delivery, assess logistics with public health and emergency management advisers, analyze supply chain capacity and operations, and determine a communications strategy. For all these efforts, GIS was foundational.

In the United States, the Department of Health and Human Services (HHS), in coordination with the Department of Defense (DoD) and the CDC, provided a strategic vaccine distribution overview and an interim plan for state, tribal, territorial, and local public health programs and their partners.

The agencies included these steps in the vaccination effort:

1. Engage with other leaders, stakeholders, and the public.

2. Distribute vaccines quickly and transparently.

3. Ensure safe vaccine administration and availability.

4. Monitor necessary data through an IT system capable of supporting and tracking distribution, administration, and other necessary data.

Outside the United States, ministries of health, nonprofit organizations, collaboratives, and consortiums espoused similar workflows. GIS became an integral part of IT systems to support vaccine distribution, engage stakeholders and the public, and provide real-time awareness and transparency.

GIS supports COVID-19 vaccine distribution in five key ways.

1. Identify facilities capable of storing and distributing the vaccine

The Pfizer and Moderna vaccines administered extensively in the United States and many other countries require cold storage, with one (initially, at least) requiring ultra-cold storage at –70 degrees Celsius. Other factors such as parking, accessibility to vulnerable populations, distance from vaccine production facilities, traffic, and overall venue size also affect which facilities can properly store and distribute a vaccine.

States surveyed their systems to identify the locations of their ultra-cold storage freezers, said Julie Swann, a professor of industrial and systems engineering at North Carolina State University, who advised the CDC. "I would expect that kind of cold storage to be available at large hospitals, scientific research facilities, and some large pharmacies."

The facilities Swann mentioned were likely those already set up for administering other vaccines in their normal course of business.

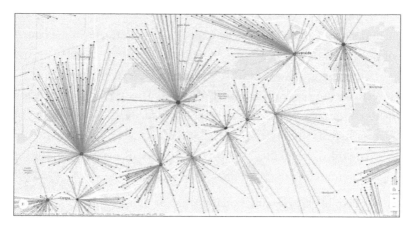

Sample vaccine venue map in which yellow dots to red dots indicate capacity for cold storage. Dot size indicates overall capacity. Lines represent drive time and distance to the venue from various population centers.

These larger, vaccine-ready facilities were selected to support phase 1 of the vaccine distribution. Because the vaccine supply was limited initially, the first priority was to vaccinate health care workers directly exposed to COVID-19 patients. The second group included essential workers who kept society running, such as police and firefighters, food packagers and distributors, and teachers and childcare providers.

A larger vaccine supply, available in phase 2 of the distribution process, required additional facilities to meet increasing demand. Sites such as private provider offices, work sites, clinics, hospitals, health departments, retail settings, and senior centers became candidates for broadening vaccine distribution. Mapping the candidate sites marked the first step to ensuring adequate population coverage.

2. Identify and prioritize critical populations

At first the vaccine was in short supply, so it was important to distribute the doses strategically and ethically. The first group, as noted, included those most likely to be exposed to COVID-19 in the course of their work.

The next group prioritized included people at increased risk for severe disease or death from COVID-19. This group included residents of nursing homes and assisted living facilities, people with risk factors such as obesity and cancer, and adults aged 65 and older.

The third group identified five categories of people at increased risk of contracting or transmitting the virus:

- People experiencing homelessness or living in shelters

- College students and workers in educational settings

- Tribal communities and members of racial and ethnic minority groups

- People living and working in crowded settings

- Incarcerated people

Health departments relied on GIS to develop a detailed view of the various priority populations and how they clustered across their jurisdictions. GIS helped pandemic responders visualize additional burdens these populations faced in receiving the vaccine, such as lack of transportation and communication barriers for non-English speakers.

Beyond visualization, it was essential for health departments to tally actual population numbers for total population and each priority group to facilitate orders of vaccine doses and estimate capacity and workforce needs in geographic context. In other words, they needed to establish how many people in each group were within 1 mile, a 15-minute walk, or a 30-minute drive of a vaccination site. GIS supported the critical match of facility capacity, vaccine supply, and population groups across locations.

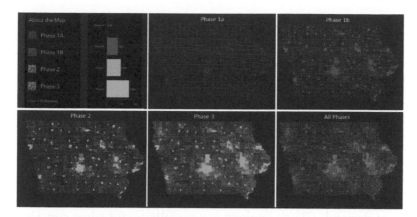

A dot density map is a useful method for showing where various populations cluster. Mapping numbers of people in priority groups for each of the COVID-19 vaccination phases offers insight to leaders as they plan vaccine distribution across their communities.

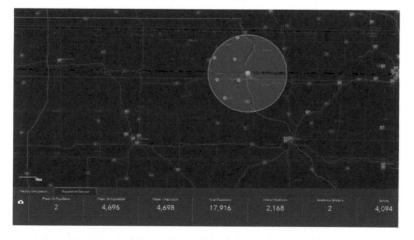

A configurable situational awareness viewer such as the one shown here can provide insights for identifying and locating new vaccine sites and determining the vaccination capacity for a proposed location.

3. Identify gaps in access and offer options for alternative distribution

After health departments identified potential vaccine distribution facilities along with critical populations to prioritize, they needed to identify potential gaps and evaluate possible solutions.

Government leaders assumed that during phase 2 of the vaccine distribution for the general population, demand would exceed the capacity of vaccination venues. To increase capacity, government leaders engaged new partners and added new vaccination sites to meet demand. GIS technology is especially useful when considering complex site location criteria, such as accessibility, population makeup, ingress and egress, budget, and more.

Furthermore, people with special needs required targeted outreach. This category included rural residents with limited access to vaccination sites, people with disabilities, underinsured and uninsured people, unhoused people, and others who were homebound or otherwise less likely to seek vaccination. GIS helped identify the most efficient routes for mobile vaccination teams.

4. Implement a vaccine management and inventory system

In the United States, guidelines for the Pfizer and Moderna vaccines initially required two doses for immunity against COVID-19, and patients were initially instructed not to interchange them. Someone receiving the Johnson & Johnson vaccine was considered fully immunized with a single dose. Then boosters were introduced, and vaccine brand crossover was allowed and sometimes encouraged. Data management became essential for vaccination records, including the dose, the brand, and the date for the next dose, as well as for monitoring and redistributing vaccines before they degraded or expired.

Health care providers and governments needed a system to capture data that quickly and accurately records individual vaccination

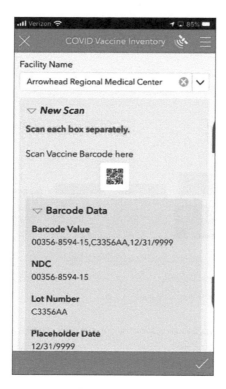

A digital survey tool can be configured to capture relevant data at the point of vaccine inventory check-in or checkout.

information, with the bar code identifying the vaccine carton and vial. The system needed to keep pace with the fast-moving vaccination process and report potential adverse reactions. In addition to tracking vaccine supply, officials also had to monitor inventories of personal protective equipment for health care workers and vaccine kits (needles, syringes, alcohol prep pads). The ArcGIS Survey123 app helped pandemic responders collect this data from a smartphone or tablet. The app read 2D bar codes for fast and accurate data entry. From there, a web-based dashboard gave decision-makers a real-time view of the constantly changing situation.

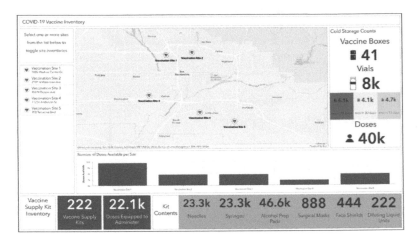

Submitted inventory counts can be tallied in real-time dashboards to enhance situational awareness and support decision-making, such as redistributing vaccine doses locally.

5. Provide transparency and accurate communication

Early transparency inspires trust and provides critical information about how and why vaccination resources are allocated in each community. ArcGIS Hub[SM] was built specifically as a community engagement platform, offering access to data, maps, and apps related to a designated initiative. An ArcGIS Hub site for COVID-19 can provide a vaccination locator service, allowing people to find key information about nearby vaccine venues.

Beyond communication to the general public, government leaders must consider targeted outreach to special populations, such as people who are wary of the vaccines or have nontraditional preferences for receiving information. Esri Tapestry[TM] Segmentation data meshes demographic data with socioeconomic, psychographic, and spending behavior data. The data offers unique insights into US neighborhoods and helps officials learn more about the needs and communication preferences of a population. Added to maps, charts,

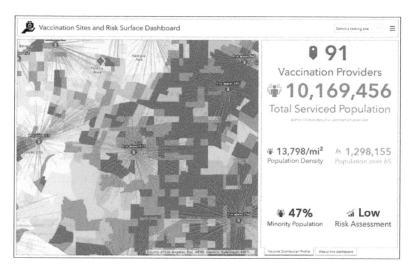

A dashboard gives stakeholders and the public an up-to-date and transparent view of the current status of the vaccination effort.

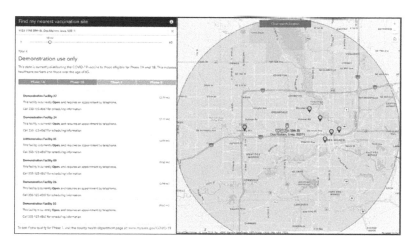

The app helps residents find vaccination venues nearest to them.

and reports, Tapestry Segmentation data can help deliver relevant and effective messages to these communities.

Conclusion

Governments and responding organizations around the world considered many factors as they developed plans for distributing the vaccine. Health responders relied on a GIS technology platform to prepare, implement, and manage COVID-19 vaccine distribution. They learned to handle communication with clarity and transparency to drive an effective vaccination campaign and strengthen public confidence in the vaccine distribution process.

A version of this story by Este Geraghty originally appeared as "How GIS Can Help Leaders Achieve Equitable, Speedy Vaccine Distribution" on the *Esri Blog* on September 24, 2020.

APPLYING LOCATION INTELLIGENCE TO VACCINE DISTRIBUTION

City of Bethlehem Health Bureau, Pennsylvania; Kansas Department of Health and Environment; and Lewis and Clark Public Health, Montana

AFTER THE APPROVAL OF TWO COVID-19 VACCINES IN December 2020, US states had to develop plans for distribution. The work started with determining who would receive the first doses in a context of limited vaccine supply, overwhelmed and overcrowded hospitals, and a shortage of staff to administer shots.

In Pennsylvania, Kansas, and Montana, health officials used geospatial technology to centralize key information, map vaccine sites, and analyze data to plan an efficient, equitable rollout.

Mapping local intention to take the vaccine in Pennsylvania

When Pennsylvania's Bethlehem Health Bureau received its first shipment of the vaccine for Northampton County, staff set up vaccine clinics, communicated with residents, targeted eligible priority groups, and determined how many more doses to order. Sherri Penchishen, Health Bureau director of Chronic Disease programs for the City of Bethlehem, rallied her COVID-19 vaccination team to create dashboards and a survey. Mapping county data with GIS has played a critical role in distribution, giving Penchishen and everyone involved a holistic view of the situation.

To gauge local intentions to take the vaccine, Penchishen and her team created a community survey using ArcGIS Survey123. The team fed survey data into smart maps, where it could be visualized to guide the Health Bureau in determining the size of vaccine clinics and deciding how much vaccine to order.

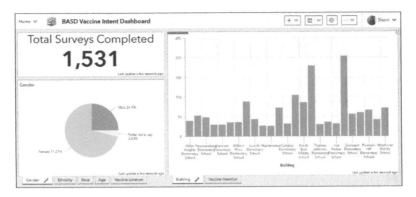

Dashboard displays the number of completed vaccine intent surveys collected by the Bethlehem Health Bureau, shown by gender and vaccine location.

Bethlehem had indoor centers and outdoor drive-through locations. Potential vaccine sites needed to accommodate an organized, efficient flow of people from registration through vaccine stations.

Penchishen and her team also created a GIS dashboard to show the number of people vaccinated and number of doses administered by every clinic; a dashboard map showed the locations of vaccine recipients. Penchishen added the second dose count to let the public know how many people had completed the series.

Another dashboard was created to inform the public of available vaccine sites, showing the number of open clinics and available doses at each site.

"Geospatial data is important in this endeavor to assure all pockets of the population are identified and the vaccine is distributed in a timely fashion," Penchishen said.

Reaching rural populations in Kansas

Throughout the COVID-19 pandemic, the GIS team at the Kansas Department of Health and Environment (KDHE) helped drive public awareness by creating maps of local cases and testing sites. When KDHE received its first vaccine shipments, the GIS team was tasked with helping to quantify the population that would be prioritized for doses.

"Because of the unknown factors in the allocation of doses, which is determined through the federal system, the vaccine staff needed a very quick and flexible manner to view the populations for priority vaccinations," said Nolita LaVoie, a GIS database specialist at KDHE.

In response, the GIS team built a dashboard using ArcGIS Dashboards, hosted in an ArcGIS Hub site that became a centralized resource for scenario planning. Vaccine staff used the GIS dashboard to locate priority populations and run scenarios for specific counties or groups. Having this information ensured that distribution strategies accounted for many variables, key to encouraging residents' participation.

State planners faced the challenge of reaching the nearly 26 percent of Kansans who live in rural areas. Since the initial vaccine

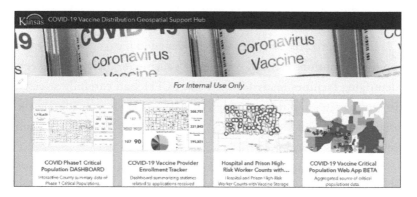

Several dashboards created by the Kansas Department of Health and Environment contain sensitive data used for scenario planning. These dashboards can be restricted for internal use only.

required ultra-cold storage and significant storage space, planners prepositioned the vaccine at select locations until it could be redistributed broadly across rural and urban locations. Using the GIS dashboards, the immunization team selected locations and vaccine redistribution routes with the goal of reaching high-risk health care workers and then others, regardless of location.

"It's tough to overstate the impact that geography has on vaccine distribution," said Amy Roust, geospatial database administrator at KDHE. "You never want someone's physical location to be a disadvantage when it comes to equitable access to health care."

Driven to make transparent decisions in Montana

In Helena, Montana, the Lewis and Clark Public Health (LCPH) department made data-driven decisions and proactively built an efficient process for vaccinating its more than 69,000 residents.

"We want to make decisions with transparency about priority groups and the challenges we face as a county with opening vaccine access up to everyone," said Tom Richardson, pharmacy clinical manager with St. Peter's Health and a member of the Lewis and Clark County vaccination team.

LCPH partnered with key stakeholders and local agencies for the rapid distribution of the 975 doses of vaccine it received per week, identifying facilities ready for the task. LCPH staff carefully selected dispensing sites and drive-through or mobile clinics, considering the particular needs of the community, including mobility challenges and limited access to technology.

"Given the issues with limited vaccine supply, our local vaccine planning team has always understood the importance of being prepared for today and this week," said Eric Merchant, former administrator of the health department's Disease Control and Prevention division. "We have built capacity by establishing more than adequate points of dispensing (POD) infrastructure and staffing."

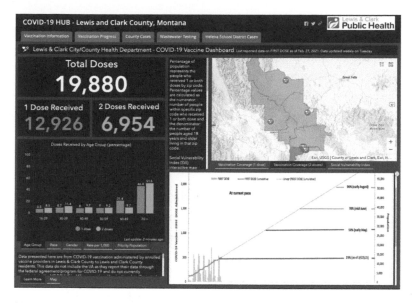

Mapping progress on vaccine distribution includes a projection of milestones met based on the current pace of vaccinations.

The LCPH team used the ArcGIS Coronavirus Vaccine Outreach solution to create a vaccine distribution information website. The site became a one-stop source of information related to community vaccine activities, including tracking vaccine recipients and their locations. The team used US Census data to estimate the percentage of population that had received the vaccine by county postal code, said Dorota Carpenedo, LCPH epidemiologist. The map displays the data for quick review.

The communication hub site features maps to give county and health department officials a real-time picture of what's going on in their area so they can make decisions accordingly. County officials can use the hub site to prioritize communities that have historically faced inequities.

"We display this information via an interactive mapping application, visualizing the vaccination reach for the first and second doses administered. This allows us to assess vaccination gaps in rural communities or communities that may be disadvantaged because of various economic factors," Carpenedo said. "Just like in other parts of the country, Montana's data clearly shows that people of color—specifically Native American and Alaska Native, and Native Hawaiian and Pacific Islander—have been disproportionately impacted by COVID-19, with higher rates of morbidity, mortality, and transmission."

Health officials can respond to these and other disparities by developing strategies to ensure equity in the availability of medical resources, including testing sites, vaccines, acute care, guidance on disease prevention, and more.

"We feel the importance of geospatial data is in our ability to show results," said Eric Spangenberg, GIS coordinator for Lewis and Clark County. "Showing the numbers on a map has an immediate impact on the reader."

A version of this story by Christopher Thomas originally appeared as "Local Agencies Apply Location Intelligence to COVID-19 Vaccine Distribution" on the *Esri Blog* on March 11, 2021.

DASHBOARDS MARK PROGRESS OF RAPID VACCINATIONS

Chilean National System for the Coordination of Territorial Information

CHILE ACHIEVED ONE OF THE QUICKEST DISTRIBUTIONS OF COVID-19 vaccines in the world. By mid-April 2021, more than 50 percent of the population had received at least one shot, well beyond any other Latin American country and behind only a few countries elsewhere in the world.

Chilean epidemiologists credit this rapid response to the country's network of clinics—placed even in the most remote regions—and its modern information infrastructure that receives input from every community.

"We incorporated the concept of territorial intelligence to share data with partners and the general population so they can make better-informed decisions," said Cristián Araneda, executive secretary for the Chilean National System for the Coordination of Territorial Information.

During the pandemic, the information system gained importance because it spans all ministries as a permanent mechanism for institutional coordination. A regular meeting led by Julio Isamit, former minister of National Assets, convened to discuss the status of COVID-19 across all territories and to share Ministry of Health data. A team of analysts created the country's COVID-19 case index and vaccination index to analyze and present this data to the various ministries to gauge impacts and guide policy.

The information system team also worked to share COVID-19 updates with the public. The team first created the COVID-19 dashboard as a way to see and share infection rates and then quickly pivoted to track progress on vaccine distribution with the *Yo Me Vacuno* ("I get vaccinated") dashboard.

"The first thing we asked ourselves was, 'Why, what is the purpose of the dashboards?'" Araneda said. "Our goal is keeping the public informed on progress and giving citizens a tool to make decisions. We want to be transparent and improve the quality of life. We also want to share good news, such as with our elderly population who are so happy after getting vaccinated, they feel as if they have another chance at life. Now in Chile, the population has the same information that the president of Chile and the minister of health have to make decisions about the pandemic."

Establishing territorial intelligence

The National System for the Coordination of Territorial Information, also known as IDE Chile *(La Infraestructura de Datos Geoespaciales de Chile)*, is the spatial data infrastructure organization that established a data exchange mechanism and optimized the management of geospatial information in Chile. IDE Chile includes many datasets regarding people, energy, environment, transportation, natural resources, government property, and disaster response. Every managed dataset in the system contains the foundational element of location to be visualized and analyzed as layers on a map using GIS. The IDE Chile team aggregated the data so it could spend more time analyzing the information and getting public buy-in.

"Our territorial intelligence policy is intended to get us closer to the population," Araneda said. "We are very technical, but we know that maps can tell a better story than raw data and present the information in a way that makes it easy for the general public to absorb and understand."

With the COVID-19 crisis, IDE Chile helped the Ministry of National Assets become a trusted source for public guidance,

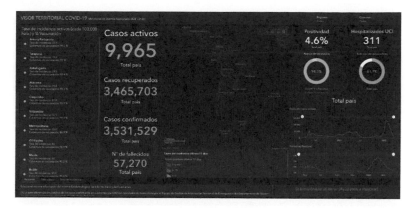

The COVID-19 dashboard in Chile is regularly presented on television so viewers can see and understand infection rates.

allowing everyone to see infection rates and vaccine management and distribution. As of late spring 2021, the COVID-19 dashboard had already received more than 4 million visits in a country of more than 19 million people. The dashboard approach has been successful with the public, politicians, and the media.

"Today, it's not uncommon to see the president making decisions using the COVID-19 dashboard or talking about the dashboard on television," Araneda said. "Every week, we can watch famous doctors on TV presenting information and drawing conclusions with the dashboard in the background."

For every initiative, IDE Chile takes great care to present the data correctly and make the tools easy to understand.

"We run a validation step with people who are not GIS specialists to make sure users can understand the details at a single glance," Araneda said. "I also want to emphasize the importance of our multidisciplinary approach to gain a variety of perspectives and to avoid reworking a project at the final stage. We have a well-tuned development process, like any R&D center, that allows us to achieve quick implementation."

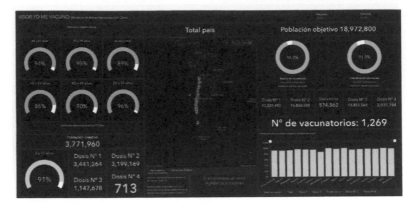

Chile's *Yo Me Vacuno* ("I get vaccinated") dashboard tracks progress on vaccine distribution and vaccination rates.

Vaccination campaign

In preparation for vaccinations, team analysts first used GIS to determine the location of vaccination sites. The vaccination team could look at sites and data on a map to consider such questions as how to reach the most people and how to make access easy for the public, factoring in the location of metro stops.

Next, the team created the *Yo Me Vacuno* dashboard to inform the public about the progress of the vaccination campaign and provide a map to guide people to vaccination hubs. Just 10 days later, the team was receiving, processing, and launching the data for public use.

"Showing the vaccination hubs helps the public make fast decisions," Araneda said. "It gives people official up-to-date information without confusion, so people can go to their nearest vaccination center, for example."

Response to the *Yo Me Vacuno* dashboard has been measured in a more qualitative than quantitative way. Rather than views of the dashboard, IDE Chile has been tracking public sentiment.

"We have seen comments on social media and our website, such as 'Thanks to this dashboard I have been able to get a vaccine quickly and safely,'" Araneda said. "People are taking the time to let us know it has had a positive impact on their lives."

Sharing national information

During the pandemic, the team put together many dashboards on other topics such as which national parks or small businesses were open at the time.

"Without a doubt, awareness of GIS has grown during this crisis," Araneda said. "Various government departments and nongovernmental organizations are getting in touch with us to set up more systems because they now understand how important these systems, maps, and dashboards have become."

Agencies and other groups are discussing ideas for future dashboards, such as systems for firefighters or for tracking environmental issues, and maps for children. The team's efforts have been recognized inside and outside the country.

"Recently, the ambassador of Peru had a meeting with the minister, and one of the main points of the conversation was how to replicate the dashboard in Peru based on the Chilean experience," Araneda said.

A version of this story by Este Geraghty originally appeared as "COVID-19: Chile Achieves Rapid Vaccinations with Dashboards Marking Progress" on the *Esri Blog* on May 13, 2021.

USING GIS TO REACH HOMEBOUND RESIDENTS FOR COVID-19 VACCINATION

Oregon Public Health Department

RETURNING TO NORMALCY AFTER THE COVID-19 PANDEMIC is everyone's goal, and vaccinations are key while moving to the next phases of economic recovery. Two barriers remain in the effort to vaccinate everyone. First, officials must encourage people who resist the vaccine to participate. Second, officials must reach the most vulnerable populations: the immobile and homebound individuals who need the vaccination brought to them.

In Clackamas County, the Oregon Public Health Department implemented a strategy to vaccinate homebound residents. Meeting the county's target of vaccinating 70 percent of its residents was critical for the county and for moving the state forward. Clackamas County is the third-most populous county in the state of Oregon, with more than 400,000 residents and an area of 1,883 square miles.

County leaders recognized the need for a solution that supported a data-driven approach to reaching their homebound population. They needed to know where vaccination requests originated and the proximity of those residents to staff and vaccination supplies. Realizing the need to connect resources to the people who needed them, pandemic responders relied on GIS technology for support. Local and county government health officials developed an operations dashboard with logistics support that helped management understand its daily tasks, improving efficiency by more than 50 percent. "Through the use of Esri's ArcGIS software, we were able to reduce the time of in-home vaccinations, which was expected to take six months, down to three months," said Kim LaCroix, public health program manager at Clackamas County.

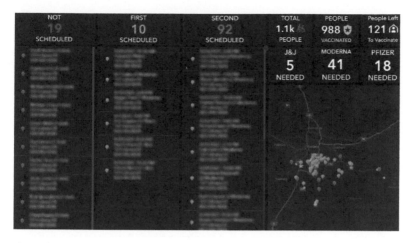

The in-home vaccination operations dashboard helps visualize key statistics in the data (names blurred for publication).

Deciding on and implementing a GIS workflow

When Clackamas County announced its in-home vaccination program, hundreds of people responded. Initially, residents received an email with a link to sign up, but the volume of requests became unmanageable. Scheduling appointments was difficult, and there was no way of visualizing appointment locations. Also, the appointment locations were far apart, all over the county, which was inefficient, cost valuable time, and led to vaccine doses going to waste. Staff tracked and monitored the vaccination requests via email and through spreadsheets but soon found the manual approach unsustainable. The county needed a solution that focused on the whereabouts of staff and resources.

Through collaboration with medical professionals, scheduling assistants, technical staff, management, public and government affairs personnel, and Esri staff, the county created an effective GIS solution. County staff used ArcGIS Survey123, a mobile-friendly survey app that gathers data, to input appointment requests, generating

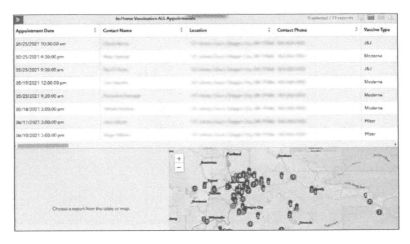

The in-home vaccination app assists with scheduling and helps nurses update patient data and vaccination details, including appointment date, name, location, phone number (blurred for publication), and type of vaccine.

a location on a web map with all the necessary patient information. The app allowed schedulers to organize vaccination requests based on location. They used ArcGIS Workforce, a mobile app solution that uses location to coordinate a field workforce, to plan daily routes for nurses.

Each day, nurses updated appointment details, navigated to appointments through their smartphones, and provided real-time information to managers to track the outcome of each home vaccination request from beginning to end. Whereas the previous workflow had required too much clerical work to constantly update information, the new GIS-enabled workflow automatically updated data from various teams and applications.

Reaching a vaccination goal in record time

Health officials must track an immense amount of data from the moment a vaccination request is entered to when a patient receives their dose. This data is summarized in a dashboard created using ArcGIS, with an interactive web map that presents location-based data on a single screen. Management staff can refresh their dashboard anytime to analyze staffing needs and communicate project status. The dashboard provides relevant information, such as the appointment date and type of vaccine, so staff can filter for the information they need.

Health officials credit the use of the geographic approach for the success of the program in reaching its goal 50 percent faster than initially expected.

The pilot program had many built-in efficiencies that led to achieving goals and performing ahead of schedule. Staff and patients felt more comfortable with the process, which in turn allowed the program to grow. Nurses and scheduling assistants adapted quickly to the new technology and integrated GIS solutions with their daily tasks. Equipping nurses with Survey123 app forms on smartphones and devices took little or no training. The decreased staff time, increase in completed appointments, and reduction of unused vaccines demonstrated the project's return on investment.

This innovation and success showed how Clackamas County improved COVID-19 vaccine distribution. As these results suggest, GIS capabilities can support vaccine effort in counties nationwide, including vaccine delivery to underrepresented communities. The COVID-19 pandemic amplified the need for integrating technology with public health through the use of critical data and analysis to ensure that every community is supported and protected.

A version of this story originally appeared as "Oregon Health Officials Use GIS to Reach Homebound Residents for COVID-19 Vaccination" on esri.com in 2021.

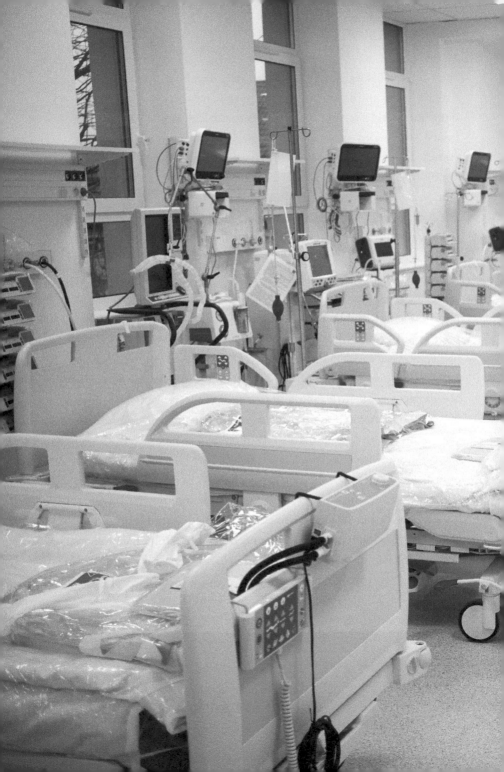

PART 3

CAPACITY AND INFRASTRUCTURE

So far in this book, we've underscored the importance of gaining situational awareness in an emergency. Part 1 highlighted that when you know where things happen in space and time, you can better comprehend the situation, predict the future, and make decisions. Deciding how to protect people at risk is often one of the first decisions that health professionals make. Part 2 emphasized the value of deploying geoenabled data and methods to identify the most vulnerable populations. During a pandemic, vulnerability leading to greater risk of illness may result from increased exposure, such as working in a service job; amplified transmission risk, such as attending a crowded event; greater infection susceptibility risk, such as advanced age and certain medical comorbidities; and sociodemographic factors, such as race. We saw that identifying vulnerability and resource gaps helped clarify where goods and services should be placed to keep people well and manage their health needs.

Part 3 will focus on keeping infrastructures healthy. This effort requires an understanding of the baseline and surge capacity of our health care infrastructure at local levels and in consideration of varying local conditions. Many experts developed compartmental models to predict how the infection would spread, which, in turn, enabled them to forecast the impact on the health

MODELS AND MAPS EXPLORE COVID-19 SURGES AND CAPACITY

Penn Medicine's Predictive Healthcare Team

EPIDEMIOLOGISTS WATCHED WITH GROWING CONCERN IN 2020 as the number of people diagnosed with COVID-19 kept increasing. As the epidemic evolved into a global pandemic, hospitals faced anticipated shortages of beds, ventilators, supplies, and medical workers.

Ahead of inquiries from concerned leaders, scientists began creating analytical models to quantify and predict the surge in COVID-19 cases. From that effort, many models emerged as predictive tools for preserving health care capacity.

Penn Medicine's Predictive Healthcare Team adapted the susceptible, infected, and recovered (SIR) mathematical model, to create a new model called CHIME (COVID-19 Hospital Impact Model for Epidemics). CHIME provided up-to-date estimates on the number of people who would need hospital care and, of that number, how many would need ICU beds and ventilators. CHIME also considered how social distancing policies might impact disease spread.

Public health administrators, hospital administrators, and government authorities from around the world quickly saw the need for forecasting models like CHIME to guide public policy and plan hospital response.

Integrated within GIS

At the onset of the COVID-19 outbreak, Esri's spatial statistics software development team incorporated several open-source models into a geospatial toolbox, starting with the CHIME model. Bringing a model into GIS aligns it directly to the data source that drives the model. This integration provides the means to visualize a problem

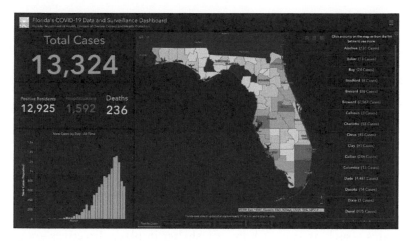

The Florida Department of Health created a dashboard to share information about cases, test results, and hospitalizations from each county across the state. Hospitalizations are an important input into the CHIME forecasting model.

geographically and ties model outputs to solutions designed for immediate and targeted action.

GIS allows deeper analysis of specific geographies to see model outputs alongside other spatially varying data, such as more vulnerable senior populations, to explore what the model results mean for people and places. This approach leads to the next question: Where and when should resources be moved or expanded to meet the demand? Tools such as location-allocation can guide those decisions and ensure that demand is met as effectively and equitably as possible.

Incorporating CHIME within GIS directly supports discussions within emergency operations centers that can display model outputs on large screens to guide collaborative planning. Then, when the time comes to decide on actions, GIS provides the means to push data and directives into map-driven apps and solutions for use in the field.

Diving into the model

Within GIS, users connect to the data sources that inform the CHIME model. This data includes current case information about the number of people hospitalized. It also includes the susceptible population and characteristics of the virus, such as the hospitalization rate and the time it takes for that rate to double.

To gain a localized forecast, GIS users can choose a specific start date and the average number of days of infection to project the current pattern forward. Many models that emerged in response to the pandemic, including CHIME, included social distancing measures—such as stay-at-home or shelter-in-place directives—and accounted for how reducing physical contact slowed the spread of the disease. To include a variable representing social distancing, modelers can use aggregated and anonymized cell phone mobility data.

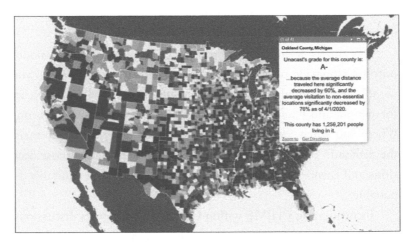

Data on mobility compares social distancing efforts to a prepandemic time as shown here with data from Unacast. Including mobility data as a parameter can help inform the forecasting models with a more accurate understanding of the varying spatial and temporal patterns of social distancing compliance.

This spatially and temporally varying input gauges social contact from high to low across an area.

Details such as average hospital stay and percentage of people who require ventilator support or intensive care are also key inputs to the model. This data can then be compared with current hospital capacity, such as available beds and ventilators. Comparing the anticipated peak of disease spread to predicted drains on hospital capacity helps local authorities plan ahead to add more hospital beds to address anticipated spikes in demand. Users can input generalized parameters (averaged over space and time) into a model. But the models will provide more accuracy and greater value if users input more precise spatial and temporal values that better represent each focus area's underlying population characteristics and social distancing behaviors.

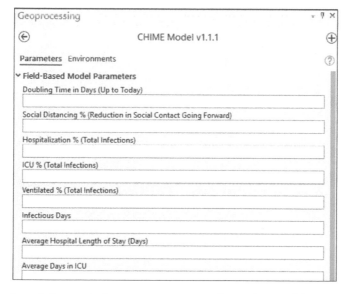

Users have full control of parameter settings in the CHIME model geoprocessing tool within ArcGIS Pro.

Visualizing policy impacts

When policy makers use a model that can tune a set of parameters to show how the forecast changes, they can examine a variety of scenarios—such as social distancing on a scale of none to stay-at-home orders. Seeing how behavior affects the course of the disease across space and time drives home the importance of policy actions during a pandemic.

Visualization of the model outputs illustrates what it means to flatten the curve. With greater social distancing, the peak (highest impact on hospital capacity) comes later with a lower and wider curve, decreasing or at least evening out the burden on medical care providers and the health care system.

Using GIS, officials can further explore the modeled forecast and answer other location-specific questions crucial to response and recovery. Pandemic responders can use the spatial analytical capabilities of GIS to analyze and answer a variety of critical questions

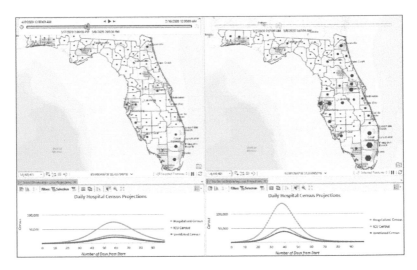

Visualizing the impact of different levels of adherence to social distancing helps authorities make difficult policy decisions.

related to COVID-19, guiding actions to reduce the impact on individuals, businesses, and health care systems.

The Esri spatial statistics software development team continues to build more models into the toolset because they believe that the more ways officials can look at the COVID-19 pandemic and its repercussions, the more prepared they will be to respond effectively.

A version of this story by Lauren Bennett and Este Geraghty originally appeared as "Models and Maps Explore COVID-19 Surges and Capacity to Help Officials Prepare" on the *Esri Blog* on April 7, 2020.

USING MAPS AND MODELS TO CREATE SURGE HOSPITAL CAPACITY

US Army Corps of Engineers

I N MARCH 2020, THE AMERICAN HOSPITAL ASSOCIATION predicted that if the curve of infection did not flatten, the need for hospital beds would exceed capacity by more than 270 percent for inpatient care and about 500 percent for intensive care.

Under its national disaster plan, the Federal Emergency Management Agency (FEMA) asked the US Army Corps of Engineers (USACE) to work with states to build and inspect alternate care facilities to augment health care capacity. A USACE team developed engineering plans for converting existing facilities with rooms (such as hotels and college dormitories) and those with large open areas (such as field houses and convention centers). From there, the team developed standardized designs and used mobile applications to assess candidate sites and inspect retrofitted facilities for readiness.

"We're looking at some amazing analytics to be able to figure out where we see the growth of the threat and where we see the bed shortage," said Lieutenant General Todd Semonite, USACE commanding general, at a White House press briefing. The team relied on spatial modeling to determine the best locations to build, he said.

As of June 2020, USACE had completed 1,155 site assessments of potential alternative care facilities across the country and constructed or modified 34 facilities, creating an additional 15,074 beds to meet the surge of seriously ill patients.

"There's really no end in sight for COVID-19, and we're going to need to continue to maintain these additional beds for some time to come," said Julie Vicars, a USACE Common Operating Picture (uCOP) manager.

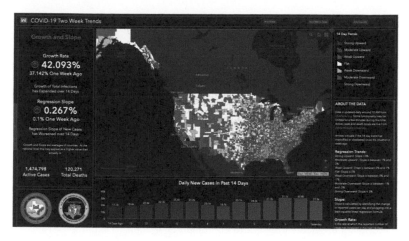

USACE's COVID-19 Two Week Trends dashboard showing growth rate of infections and regression slope of new cases. This static image was captured on June 22, 2020.

Models show where capacity is needed most

The USACE modeling and analysis team analyzed several models used in the coronavirus pandemic. Many epidemiologists adapted the long-standing susceptible, exposed, infected, and recovered (SEIR) models for COVID-19. For example, Columbia University created a spatiotemporal transmission model that predicted the spread of infections across China before turning to a global view. The Institute for Health Metrics and Evaluation (IHME) at the University of Washington used modeling to project the locations and number of cases and deaths. Penn Medicine's Predictive Healthcare Team created the COVID-19 Hospital Impact Model for Epidemics, or CHIME. The Center for Army Analysis and the US Army Engineer Research and Development Center conducted daily modeling efforts.

"General Semonite wanted to know why all of a sudden there were five models," said Rick Vera, the geospatial branch chief at USACE's Galveston district and team lead for the modeling effort.

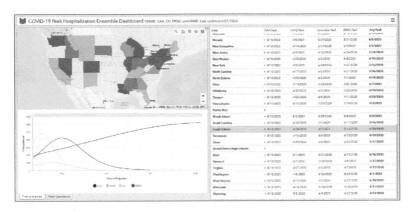

The original ensemble dashboard combined all models to explore and see how different scenarios might play out.

"Colonel David Hibner, commander of the US Army Geospatial Center, had the idea of putting them all together, kind of like a spaghetti model, so that all models could be looked at in one graph to see which were more optimistic and to see which ones predicted that the peak cases would extend into late summer or even fall."

The modeling and analysis team consisted of an *ad hoc* grouping of geospatial experts from several USACE offices, working remotely. This team hosted its dashboards and analyses on USACE's enterprise GIS application. Together the team gathered model outputs into an ensemble dashboard using ArcGIS Insights[SM], which allowed this team and the rest of USACE and its federal partners to view the analyses for decision-making.

"We're moving into a very robust dashboard that allows us to slice and dice all of the models at the state and county levels," Vera said. "We can look at ICU bed predictions across all models rather than one-off queries for each model."

In April 2020, there were varied projections of the peak of the virus and the impact of social distancing. To take early, decisive action, USACE leadership needed accurate data and analyses quickly.

"We started to model the geography and to create a time series hot spot map, and that changed everything," Vera said.

Within a week, the team developed tools that helped put capacity decisions in motion for alternate care facilities. The team members added daily updates to reflect current realities and ensure clean data. Vera said the team was also "providing more analytical products for people to ingest and create their own maps, web apps, and dashboards."

With increasing numbers of dashboards displaying case counts, the USACE modeling team recognized the need to shift the view away from what had happened toward what was happening.

"We started thinking about new ways to slice and dice the data," said Jason Jordan, a GIS analyst in the Geospatial Branch in USACE's Galveston District. "We have a script that pulls daily historical data from USAfacts.org and calculates the infection growth rate and linear regression trend of new cases over the last 14 days. This gives us a timeline and a summary of the current data compared to how it was before. Immediately, we can see if things are getting better or worse and at what intensity. The dashboard also allows users to filter by states, divisions, districts, metro areas, office commuting areas, and individual counties so the decision-makers can zoom in on their area of interest."

Tools for alternate care facility site inspectors

At the start of the effort to determine suitable facilities, individual states used spreadsheets to gather criteria for potential sites. Collecting data from spreadsheets quickly became an unwieldy way to manage large amounts of tabular information as the number of potential sites increased. This process could have slowed the inspection process.

A small team of USACE geospatial professionals devised an app using ArcGIS Survey123. The team created a standard survey that

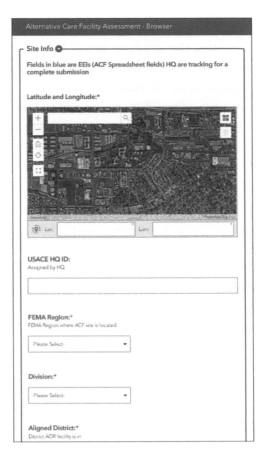

A simple survey form was created using ArcGIS Survey 123 to gather details and assess each candidate alternative care facility site.

inspectors used, with little or no training, to collect data about alternate care facilities during field inspections. The form-based app captured details such as the number of stairwells, the condition of the HVAC system, a facility's proximity to active hospitals, concerns about the existence of hazardous waste, and more. The collected data fed into a web-based editor that populated a dashboard, providing an enterprise view of facilities nationwide.

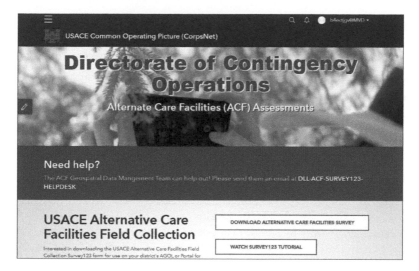

A centralized website offered answers to questions about the field survey tool and guided the facilities field data collection effort.

"Once it was established and some guidance went out, districts ran with it with no training," said Vicars, who helped lead the inspection effort. "It was feet to the fire, because the majority using it had little to no experience with the geospatial world."

At the height of assessment efforts, an average of 450 people per day used the Survey123 data collection app to gather details about potential sites. After the initial site assessment, USACE prepared the selected sites for contracting and construction. The geospatial team then added fields in Survey123 to capture additional data and further guide site development. Preparation work included adding nurse stations, installing call buttons, and piping oxygen to each room.

"Teams would go out to conduct these assessments and you would have a civil engineer looking at one piece, a structural engineer looking at another piece, and an environmentalist looking at another piece," Vicars said. "Each would add bits of information based on their subject matter expertise."

Enterprise GIS in support of capacity success

An enterprise geospatial infrastructure powered the forecast models and assessments as the pandemic pushed USACE to a new level of enterprise integration. USACE engaged its 52 districts to collect and share data during the crisis.

Hospital beds across the country were readied as a safety net for a COVID-19 surge or other disaster as USACE stepped up to its mission of providing engineering solutions for our nation's toughest challenges.

A version of this story by Ben Conklin originally appeared as "COVID-19: Army Corps Uses Maps and Models to Create Surge Hospital Capacity" on the *Esri Blog* on June 23, 2020.

SOLVING MEDICAL SUPPLY CHAIN PROBLEMS

Direct Relief

I N EARLY 2020, THE AID ORGANIZATION DIRECT RELIEF received reports about a hospital in Wuhan, the capital of China's Hubei province, describing depleted supplies of masks, gloves, and other personal protective equipment (PPE).

"That was really unusual because China makes most of the PPE," said Andrew Schroeder, Direct Relief's vice president of research and analysis. "We thought, well, if they are having a problem, this could be a really big issue."

Direct Relief, based in Santa Barbara, California, specializes in solving supply chain problems during emergencies. When disasters strike, the organization determines the best way to obtain needed supplies, often working with private manufacturers to direct products to relief zones.

As the severity of the COVID-19 outbreak increased, Direct Relief helped 50 institutions in five Chinese cities acquire masks, gloves, and other PPE. Direct Relief staff used its GIS to map and analyze the flow of goods to determine who needed supplies and where.

"Because we don't normally work in China, there were a lot of questions coming up as to where the supply was required," Schroeder said. "It was essential to begin creating basic GIS dashboards to show who needed what and where we were shipping."

Tracking the pandemic

As the outbreak spread globally, the Direct Relief team knew that the United States would get hit hard.

"We work throughout the US, primarily with community health centers and free clinics, so we began reaching out to understand what their needs were," Schroeder said. "We got really concerned this would be a major issue, so we began refocusing around stockpiles of PPE."

The pandemic spread quickly across the country, overwhelming hospitals. Health centers and clinics struggled to handle the overflow. Lacking enough PPE to keep their staff safe, several centers considered shutting down.

Breaking bottlenecks

By March 2020, Direct Relief had redirected its COVID-19 efforts to the United States. From a supply chain perspective, the problem was as much of a once-a-century event as the pandemic itself.

"We were just trying to figure out a way to deal with the increasing bottleneck on the supply chain," Schroeder said. "We'd never responded to an event like this, where all of a sudden everybody needed the same things at the same time. And supply networks just aren't set up to deal with that."

In places like New York, the pandemic forced some hospitals to devote all their resources to COVID-19 patients. But Direct Relief was also committed to helping institutions gather needed supplies and pharmaceuticals for other services.

"People don't stop having babies, getting into car accidents, or going into diabetic shock," Schroeder noted. "As people redirect resources toward the treatment of COVID-19, we have the ability to make sure there are places that are supplied for the treatment of everything else."

Just a few months after the first warnings of supplies running short in Wuhan, Direct Relief found itself in the unfamiliar position of supporting major US hospitals.

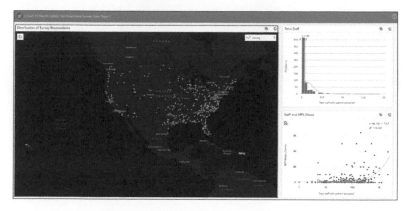

Direct Relief used ArcGIS Insights to model safety-net readiness for COVID-19 around the country by looking at the availability of staff and N95 masks.

"Given the supply chain pressures and the numbers of patients that were coming, there was a need for an all-hands-on-deck approach," Schroeder said. "To go from knowing that ICUs could be overwhelmed and that we might have to backstop folks to actually giving humanitarian support to some of the most sophisticated hospitals in the world is really crazy."

The next step

When the pandemic began, Direct Relief staff focused on managing and monitoring supply chains using GIS maps and dashboards. "GIS is part of almost everything we do," Schroeder said. "The first thing is being able to quickly start creating distribution maps that show who we're being contacted by, who we're supporting, and where the supply is going." With the continuing crisis, the organization has increasingly leaned on spatial analyses to better understand how and where to distribute services.

A version of this story by Ryan Lanclos originally appeared as "COVID-19: How Direct Relief Solves Medical Supply Chain Problems" on the *Esri Blog* on May 14, 2020.

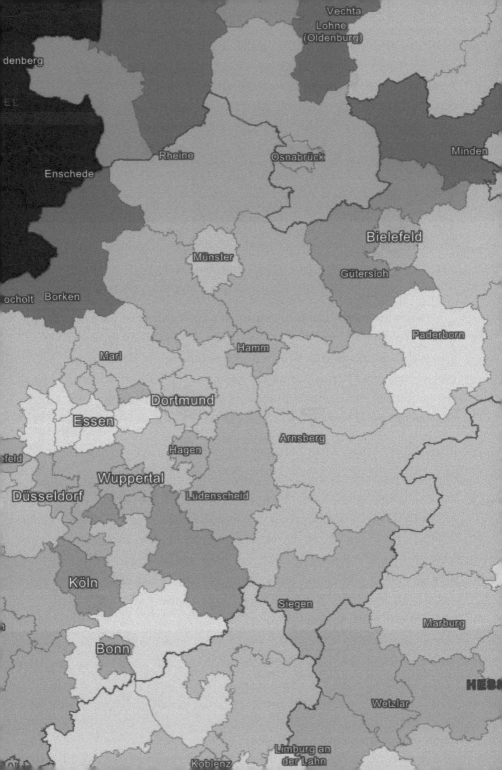

PART 4

COMMUNICATION AND ENGAGEMENT

HEALTH IS TRULY BOTH AN ART AND A SCIENCE. THE scientific aspects are perhaps obvious, evidenced by mountains of research, complex analytics, intricate technologies, and ground-breaking therapeutics. But the art of health is no less important and relies heavily on effective communication.

Health communication is "the art and technique of informing, influencing, and motivating individual, institutional, and public audiences about important health issues," according to the disease prevention campaign, Healthy People 2010. The ability to influence and motivate good health is vital in preventing disease, promoting well-being, and increasing awareness about health concerns and solutions, such as pandemic risks and resources.

Ideally, health communication is bidirectional. For instance, one might engage community members to better understand their attitudes, opinions, and needs. It can also provide data openly and effectively, allowing others to interrogate and innovate. Effective health communication extends to making interactive maps and dashboards, which allow people to see data patterns, such as the spread of COVID-19 infections in their hometown, and engage with health authorities on any number of issues. The intent, of course, is to gain increased buy-in and trust for any advice or call to action included in the messaging effort.

Successful communications require a thoughtful and comprehensive approach. First, it's essential to educate the audience on the issue being addressed. It's no simple task to reframe complex health challenges into clear, accessible, and useful information for a target audience. Sometimes, especially in public health, the audience is everyone. Reaching everyone may seem an impossible task, but we can approach that goal through geography. A geographic approach to health communication helps us understand how subgroups within a community think and behave. Using localized information, we can identify real and perceived barriers to good health and tailor disease prevention campaigns to achieve a more positive response. To this end, geography can help officials identify popular marketing channels to reach audiences and recruit credible partners to amplify the message. Geography also can help us monitor communication efforts to determine their impact. How many people are exposed to the message? Where do they live? What are their reactions? Is behavior changing in desired ways? Are adjustments necessary?

This section of the book features a variety of communication and engagement efforts that worked. You'll learn why ArcGIS Hub sites are different from regular websites and how they have helped countless organizations transparently share information, provide open data, interact with residents, and engender trust.

Earlier, we learned that part of responding to the pandemic is recognizing where vulnerabilities, risks, and needs differ across a population. The same eye toward equity is important in engagement strategy. In this section, equitable engagement is explored through the example of communities of color. This approach, which includes community health assessments and crowdsourcing, can be used for any disadvantaged group and for any community as a whole. By focusing on equitable and inclusive engagement methodologies, the health professions can advance toward their goal of lifting everyone to their best health.

The use of GIS for health communication and engagement is the theme of the next example in this section. With a large, 35-person GIS team, Cobb County, Georgia, was well positioned for the pandemic. Within days, the county provided an array of interactive maps and apps that were popular with residents, and its GIS communications hub quickly became the authoritative and reliable source for coronavirus information.

Finally, you'll learn about the efforts of the of US Census Bureau to execute the 2020 count as the pandemic grew. Although a large portion of the population responded to the organization's first-time digital questionnaires, streamlining some of the work, the Census Bureau confronted new barriers in trying to reach those considered hardest to count. Under normal circumstances, local census enumerators would visit people door-to-door to complete surveys. But would residents be receptive to interviews in a physically distanced, mask-wearing environment? Census leaders knew they had to think differently. They evaluated attitudes about home visits to inform their policies and embraced a marketing approach to engage hard-to-count individuals and families. The Census Bureau successfully pivoted when it mattered most, and now its approach—supported by research—is being tested as a way to improve confidence in COVID-19 vaccines and all other vaccines.

COMMUNICATION HUB SITES SHARE COVID-19 NEWS, RESOURCES

Montgomery County, Pennsylvania; Maryland Department of Information Technology; University of South Florida; and Delaware County, Indiana

WHILE MANY PEOPLE TUNE IN TO NEWS STORIES ABOUT the global spread of COVID-19, they also need to know how the pandemic is affecting their neighborhoods and cities.

Responding to this need, many state and local governments and agencies have created communication hub sites to share maps and information about community spread, hospital occupancy, testing stations, school closures, childcare facilities for essential workers, food banks, grocery stores, and social distancing requirements.

Even in ordinary times, communication hub sites increase transparency with the public and build trust in local governments. They have been especially important during the pandemic, allowing leaders to share current news and resources and interact with residents. Across the United States, we see hundreds of examples of communication hub sites built using ArcGIS.

Pennsylvania county monitors COVID-19 spread

Officials in Montgomery County, Pennsylvania, established its hub site when the county had its first case of COVID-19 in early March 2020. This initiative began with a visual story showing the locations of COVID-19 cases in the state and county and evolved into a full hub site with maps, resources, and pandemic information.

The ArcGIS Hub site in Montgomery County included vital information about COVID-19, symptoms, and prevention. The site also contained county-specific statistics, such as age, gender, race,

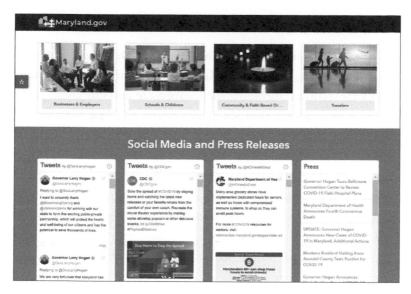

Maryland communication hub site provides an array of pandemic-related information and resources for residents and visitors.

and the municipalities of COVID-19 cases, along with local county news and updates from Governor Tom Wolf. The hub hosted public testing registration forms for residents to preregister for testing at various sites.

A stand-alone business page, accessible from the site, was created for the Montgomery County business community to share information about business loans and enable businesses to notify customers of closures or discounts.

"It's turned into an information platform with a lot of links to resources and information, especially as we've gotten more cases," said David Long, GIS manager for Montgomery County, shortly after the launch of the site in early 2020. "Our residents want to see maps and data. So, the goal of our site is to put information out in a timely manner and showcase the power of our GIS program."

Maryland opens data to instill public confidence

In just a few hours, staff from the Maryland Department of Information Technology built an ArcGIS Hub site featuring a dashboard with vital statistics, including the locations of cases by county. The site provided information about symptoms and best practices for social distancing, with links to local health departments. It included practical resources such as links to information from the CDC and resources highlighted by Governor Larry Hogan through his official website. The site also tracks current hospitalizations for COVID-19 patients, hospital capacity statewide, and other key statistics for the pandemic.

"I want to instill confidence in Marylanders that their state government is providing accurate and timely data," said Julia Fischer, director of geospatial services at the Maryland Department of Information Technology. "The data is accessible to all Marylanders and is providing a clear and definitive picture of the state's response to the unprecedented events occurring right now."

The hub, created in partnership with the Maryland Governor's Office, Maryland Emergency Management Agency, Maryland Department of Health, and other agencies, has received millions of page views since its launch in 2020.

Florida university serves open data to researchers through its communication hub site

At the University of South Florida in Tampa, Florida, a GIS team developed the Florida COVID-19 Hub site with real-time updates on a regional and statewide scale, and customized and curated applications for the Greater Tampa Bay area. The site pulls state-level data from the Florida Department of Health and global data from the Johns Hopkins University dashboard. It also archives daily datasets, shared as open data, for state, national, and international scales

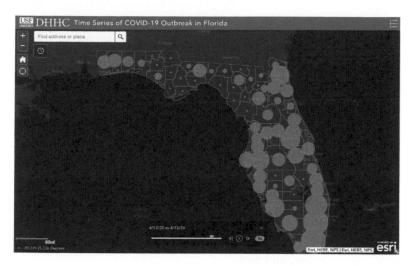

A time series application created by GIS Project Manager Benjamin Mittler shows the spread of COVID-19 across counties in Florida.

with the aim of supporting research efforts and identifying temporal trends.

The hub site has sections for statistics, social media, and custom maps displaying case counts in each Florida county, including the number of deaths, positive tests, and hospitalizations. In addition, the site provides postal code–level analysis for the Tampa Bay region. A time series application, updated automatically, shows the spread through time across counties in Florida.

"We are trying to help serve our campus researchers and engage the community of learners and educators, as well as the broader local and regional areas," said Lori Collins, research associate professor and codirector of the Digital Heritage and Humanities Center in the University of South Florida Libraries. "At this time, spatial data and its relationships to societal function and news are of vital importance."

The Florida COVID-19 site quickly received more than 400,000 views with positive public response. The site also serves university researchers by providing a spatial foundation for grant research and helping researchers connect to data, funding, and collaboration opportunities.

Indiana county creates local news site

The GIS department in Delaware County, Indiana, produced a COVID-19 ArcGIS Hub site featuring current local cases and self-reported illnesses and recoveries. Additional pages focused on vaccine distribution, food resources, testing, school closures, business and employment resources, daily briefing videos from county emergency management, and more.

The site pulls data from the Health Department and Emergency Management Agency in Delaware County, which has tracked self-reported illnesses and recoveries. It incorporates content from the Indiana Department of Health, including state maps and statistics, and summarizes information using graphs, maps, and a dashboard.

"The main purpose of our local coronavirus hub site is to be the official source for our community's response to the COVID-19 epidemic," said Kyle Johnson, coordinator for Delaware County's GIS department. "Having a one-stop shop for all the most important local information was very important to local officials and residents."

Johnson said the initial implementation in 2020 was simple, with nearly 2,000 residents accessing the site each day in the early stages of the pandemic.

A version of this story by Cassandra Perez and Maria Jordan originally appeared as "State and Local Government Open Data Sites Share COVID-19 News, Resources" on the *Esri Blog* on April 23, 2020.

EQUITABLE COMMUNITY ENGAGEMENT DURING COVID-19

Esri

COMMUNITIES OF COLOR HAVE AN ONGOING HISTORY OF being unserved or underserved with the resources they need to thrive. These circumstances tend to be magnified during times of crisis. The COVID-19 pandemic has been no different, placing communities of color at a great disadvantage, with higher risk of illness and death. Given this reality, proactive engagement is critical and must be consciously equitable.

Engage communities of color

A smart community response to a crisis is inclusive of its members at every decision-making point. To that end, the people most affected by a disaster must have a seat at the table. Including them helps ensure that the right solutions are proposed. Without community engagement, the nuances of a solution may be missed. For example, if increasing testing is the goal, it might make sense to add more testing sites. However, if the problem is not the number of sites but transportation, safety, and open hours at testing sites, simply adding sites will not help. Listening and responding to community needs offer greater insight as responders seek to connect problems with solutions. During the pandemic, organizations must engage communities of color in the planning, implementation, and recovery phases of the response. And further engagement should be part of any strategy beyond the pandemic, correcting historical inequities and helping communities thrive.

Key stages of engagement

Equitable engagement is a broad and ongoing process. However, there are a few critical moments to prioritize engagement with communities of color and other disproportionately burdened stakeholders:

- **Analysis and assessment:** Engage with communities of color in focused equity discussions when attempting to assess the impact of the crisis. Their input is essential to understanding where the needs are greatest and to make investments upstream.

- **Resource allocation planning:** Engage with communities of color when planning where and how to distribute critical resources. Doing so ensures the right resources get to the right places in the right ways.

- **Ongoing status updates:** Engage with communities of color throughout policy implementation. Getting real-time feedback may offer reassurance that the policy has had the intended impact and will provide insight about needed adjustments.

GIS can help

Esri has tools that support engagement with communities in an equitable framework to address their needs. What follows is a review of three ArcGIS applications that can be employed to facilitate equitable community engagement: ArcGIS Survey123, ArcGIS Hub, and ArcGIS StoryMaps[SM].

Survey123: Gathering community needs

The Survey123 app engages constituents and helps users learn about community needs. Surveys can be implemented in multiple ways:

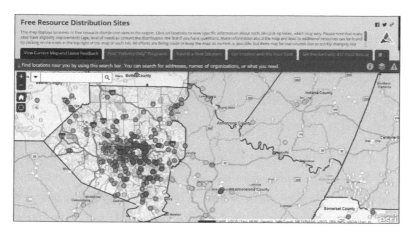

This application shows resource distribution sites across Allegheny County. The application allows viewers to search for food delivery programs, volunteer opportunities, food distribution sites, and more.

through targeted surveys, randomized community assessment surveys, and crowdsourcing data. Crowdsourcing is the process of collecting information that people volunteer. Each method can provide critical insights into a community's needs.

Allegheny County, Pennsylvania, created a crowdsourcing application for food resources in the community in response to COVID-19. The county generated a map showing food and resource distribution sites for people in need. It also provided information about how to use benefits such as the Supplemental Nutrition Assistance Program (SNAP). The county supports various ways for community members to get involved, such as volunteering for short-term events and using Survey123 to keep food resource information current. Allegheny County established formal community partnerships with the Greater Pittsburgh Community Food Bank, 412 Food Rescue, and local schools to create the most holistic picture possible of the county's resources. This collaboration has benefited all involved.

"The crowdsourced resource distribution application currently showcases 700-plus locations because of our partnerships and help from the community," said Melinda Angeles, a GIS professional for Allegheny County. "We have seen updates or new distribution locations submitted every day since launching this map to the public."

ArcGIS Hub: Partner with existing networks

As exemplified by Allegheny County, community engagement must include existing community networks. Engagement means meeting people where they live, learn, work, worship, and play. Engagement involves partnering with faith-based, educational, and community organizations. Some community partnerships may be temporary, focused on solving an immediate problem, and many others may be long-term arrangements that persistently promote and advance equity.

Hub supports collaboration through participatory engagement with community organizations, volunteers, and individual community members. When aligned and organized in a hub, the various stakeholders can provide vital insight into the needs of communities, such as access to broadband, smart technology, and personal computers. Stakeholders can also talk about the impacts of disparities on communities. Esri provides ready-to-use hub templates that users can deploy quickly in support of health equity and other initiatives associated with pandemic response. The ArcGIS Solutions website provides frequent updates.

Browse existing Hub sites

Many communities launched Hub sites in response to the pandemic, Reviewing what others have done often inspires new ideas and expanded avenues of spatial thinking. For example, the Seneca Nation Coronavirus Response Hub and the Navajo Epidemiology Center provide extensive online resources for citizens of their

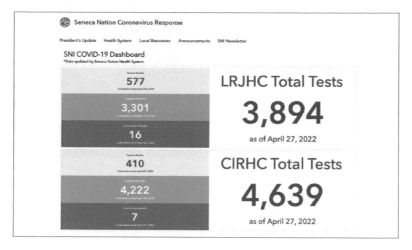

Seneca Nation's Coronavirus Response Hub, providing local resources to support the nation's community.

respective nations. Collaborating with existing entities that have experience working with underserved communities could jump-start a program, accelerating its success.

ArcGIS StoryMaps: Storytelling for health equity

Interactive stories created from ArcGIS StoryMaps technology can help communicate where and why racial and health inequities exist. Stories that embed interactive maps, text, videos, photos, and other media offer an immersive experience that can change hearts and minds and inspire action. An interactive story called *Death in Black & White* by DemLabs offers a good example. This story focuses on racial inequities in access to health care and why voting and participating in the US Census can bring about change.

A best practice for telling any story about racial or health inequities is to ensure that the people most impacted by the inequities participate in crafting the narrative.

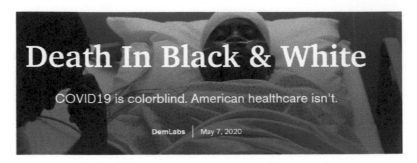

A story by DemLabs, created using ArcGIS StoryMaps, about inequities in access to health care.

Many efforts launched over the last decade or so aim to transform the health care approach into one that is more humane, inclusive, and collaborative. ArcGIS technologies such as Survey123, Hub, and ArcGIS StoryMaps readily support that transformation.

A version of this story by Rebecca Lehman, Margot Bordne, and Clinton Johnson originally appeared as "Community Engagement for Racial Equity during COVID-19" on the *ArcGIS Blog* on April 18, 2020.

GIS HUB HELPS KEEP RESIDENTS INFORMED AND SAFE

Cobb County, Georgia

W HEN AN EMERGING AND UNPREDICTABLE THREAT TO public health and safety such as the pandemic encroaches on local communities, it can be difficult for citizens to know what information they can trust and to whom they should listen.

Cobb County, Georgia, took swift, decisive action to instill confidence among its 770,000 residents using a disaster response solution from Esri. The county's COVID-19 Community Hub helps protect the local community against the spread of the coronavirus, providing authoritative, location-based data and critical resources from statewide agencies in an online platform.

Mobilizing a collaborative multiagency emergency response

The accelerating spread of COVID-19 across the country required Cobb County's GIS team to act quickly, in coordination with county management, to help safeguard the health security of their community. To do so, they needed to configure a new, centrally located, online GIS hub solution that could rapidly engage and inform their constituents, providing geospatial data and community-driven resources in near real time on interactive dashboards, smart maps, and applications.

"This pandemic is having a tremendous impact on our own community, and we want to make sure that we're addressing the current needs of our citizens," said Jennifer Lana, GIS manager for Cobb County. "We are directly supporting not just the community as a whole but our families, our neighbors, and people that we talk to

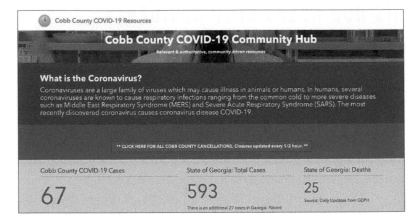

Authoritative data and community-driven resources keep local citizens informed and safe.

every day. And as this emerging threat grows, we need to be the source of authoritative data. We want them to trust us as not only the people that give the data but also as fellow community members."

The early days of the pandemic required Cobb County's 35-member GIS team to adhere to the state's shelter-in-place guidelines, which required the team to complete the workflow while working remotely.

"Because we have such a strong relationship with the county's management team, when they needed to quickly get critical information out to the public, they came directly to us," said Lana. "We had been tracking our own department data on very simple maps and posting them on a static web page. Given the escalating situation, [the management team] requested we help them share the COVID-19 data and statistics on interactive maps, because that's what everybody was asking for."

To meet the dynamic challenges, Cobb County staff prioritized GIS data in their coordinated response to the emerging public health threat. Using location intelligence, they helped keep local citizens safe, fully informed, and situationally aware. They provided data and resources visualized on interactive maps and apps in the county's COVID-19 Community Hub.

Providing a go-to destination for critical resources

As the disease outbreak spread statewide, the county's GIS department relied on ArcGIS for a template solution. The GIS department began adopting and configuring ready-to-use datasets and applications, including interactive smart maps and dashboards, to build out the county's own unique solution, the COVID-19 Community Hub.

"We really wanted to make sure our hub and the critical data in it were fully interactive for people. Our team's history of direct engagement with our local community built a foundation of trust, positioning us as a reliable data source that can be counted on in an emergency," said Lana. "So, when this situation began, we asked for feedback from the local community. Getting that direct input—whether it's via social media, email, or our crowdsourced surveys—helped inform our decision-making on what applications we needed to incorporate from Esri's COVID-19 GIS Hub, then build out and deploy."

Cobb County built and deployed its hub in two days, providing transparency into the county's coordinated pandemic response. Compatible with mobile devices, Community Hub provides near real-time data on active COVID-19 cases and fatalities at the county, state, and national scales via interactive smart maps, dashboards, and planning reports. Citizens can study the data and view current incidence by date, frequency, and severity.

Smart maps show areas with vulnerable populations, while impact-planning reports offer insights on the pandemic, including numbers, trends, and patterns. Users can access a central location for the latest news and announcements. Resources include videos, news releases, emergency orders, social media updates, and live updates from the county, state, and area schools.

"The sheer size and nature of this crisis presented the right opportunity to use all of the geospatial capabilities available in the COVID-19 GIS Hub as a central access point for monitoring and data and support," Lana said.

The Community Hub offers an array of resources:

- **The Grocery Stores hub page** distinguished Cobb County as the first local government in the country to launch an interactive map and dashboard that captured and displayed inventory levels of essential goods in individual grocery stores. Residents appreciated the ability to see what was available, and where, given shelter-in-place orders in effect at the time. The inventory data came from more than 500 shoppers who completed a crowdsourcing survey reflecting their experience. People could also see each store's social distancing guidelines and seniors-only shopping hours.

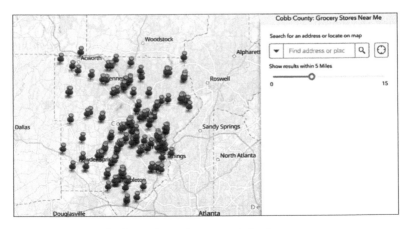

The Community Hub allowed people to search for the nearest grocery store and see its inventory of essential supplies using interactive GIS maps.

- **The Emergency and Medical Locations web map** provided the location and status of all local hospitals and medical facilities, urgent care centers, drugstores, and dialysis facilities.

- **The Food Resources interactive map** identified the locations of Cobb County School District food pickup sites, food pantries, SNAP resources, community gardens, and farmers markets.

- **The Restaurant Reporter Survey hub page** was powered by a crowdsourced survey, feeding interactive smart maps that showcase restaurant locations and pickup and delivery information.

- **The Life Is Good in Cobb County interactive story** helped locals stay connected, positive, and "share the vibe" in an interactive story. Residents could add thank-you notes, inspirational photos, and so on.

- **The COVID-19 Emergency Order application** allowed residents to report potential violations of the county's emergency declaration related to businesses, crowds, and facilities. The data collected from the Survey123 app was visualized and analyzed on an internal-only smart map for law enforcement.

Protecting the community with a map-based understanding of risk

The COVID-19 Community Hub has served as the foundation for the county's emergency communications channels, providing a transparent view of emergency response efforts. Its dashboards have captured and communicated COVID-19 data, providing a real-time, map-based understanding of community spread and evolving risk factors.

"Our new Community Hub has proven to be a very successful tool to take on this situation. The interactive capabilities of this solution give us the ability to effectively engage local citizens, which has been great," said Lana. "The mobile-friendly features and resources that it provides have allowed us to directly respond to the urgent needs of the people in our community."

Sharing location-based data detailing the scope, scale, and spread of the pandemic in near real time helps prioritize the county's emergency disaster response. Increased situational awareness and a common operating picture support collaboration, communication, and coordination among government agencies, ensuring that resources are available to save lives.

"This is obviously a very different challenge than any of us have ever experienced. The response is a lot different. It is highly personal," said Lana. "We are directly supporting our neighbors, our schools, and the local businesses and organizations all around us. It's important to recognize that while this is our job—fulfilling our roles as county employees—we also live here. We are a part of this community."

A version of this story originally appeared as "Cobb County Uses a GIS Hub to Keep Residents Informed and Safe" on esri.com in 2020.

LOCATION INTELLIGENCE HELPS BOOST CENSUS RESPONSE RATES

US Census Bureau

THE US CENSUS BUREAU FACED UNIMAGINABLE challenges with its 2020 population count, given the public health measures brought on by the pandemic. The Census Bureau curtailed typical household visits for a time until infection spikes settled and had to make difficult choices about its methods.

"In the middle of this, we had to decide whether our enumerators should wear masks," said Nancy Bates, then senior researcher for Survey Methodology at the Census Bureau. "We conducted a survey asking, 'If an enumerator comes to your door wearing a mask, would you be more likely to respond, less likely, or wouldn't it make a difference?' We found that when combined, the majority said they would prefer a mask, or it wouldn't make a difference."

The survey exemplifies the analytical approach the Census Bureau takes to assess every task, set standards, and become more efficient. For the first time, digital submissions were allowed via the internet (in addition to mail and phone responses), and the bureau used location intelligence and lifestyle segmentation data to guide its outreach. Location intelligence, or spatial intelligence, results from the analysis and visualization of geospatial data. Adding layers of geospatial data, such as traffic, weather, and the spread of infectious disease, to a smart map or dashboard can provide insights into what caused an event to happen and what might happen next.

Addressing low response rates

The US Constitution mandates a population count in each state and territory every 10 years. The results become a key metric for

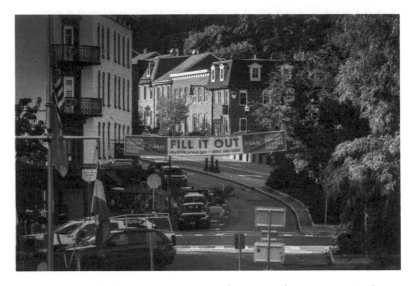

Communities, including Kingston, New York, promoted participation in the census because an accurate count translates into federal dollars for local governments to provide services.

distributing federal funds. This data influences the makeup of election districts and describes the US population at every geographic level.

Despite the importance of the data, the agency experiences low response rates from certain populations throughout the country, which can significantly limit the amount of government and commercial services they receive. The Census Bureau addresses this issue by placing ads tailored to local interests, which are determined by using location analytics. The effort reflects a quest that marketing professionals understand all too well: reaching an elusive audience.

As part of its digital transformation, the Census Bureau studied ways to improve its reach. In 2015, Census Bureau staff evaluated whether online forms improved response rates and assessed the best mix of ads and ad channels for targeting hard-to-reach residents in Savannah, Georgia. The bureau presented the results in a report called *Viewing Participation in the US Census through the Lens of Lifestyle Segments.*

The primary focus was on gaining insight into the makeup, location, and behavior of hard-to-survey populations to improve response rates among those groups. To begin that analysis, bureau staff turned to a technique popularized by marketers—lifestyle segmentation data using GIS.

Segmenting the audience

First, the Census Bureau researchers used location intelligence to derive a low response score, a metric that guided further analysis of areas determined to be the hardest to count. Then those areas were mapped and overlaid with data of each area's lifestyle segments. The Census Bureau analysis used Tapestry, a geodemographic system that integrates consumer traits with residential characteristics to identify markets, classify US neighborhoods, and depict consumer lifestyles and stages.

Derived from a combination of cluster analysis and data mining, Tapestry groups together neighborhoods with the most similar characteristics. After analyzing and correlating nonresponders to these groups, Census Bureau staff performed deeper analysis to find outreach opportunities, just as a corporate marketing team might.

Using the location intelligence generated by GIS, the Census Bureau correlated areas of historically low census response with the locations of various population segments to identify those that most needed outreach. The six population segments with the lowest participation rates had similar characteristics: they were renters, single-person households, and people with high mobility, low education, low income, and limited fluency in English.

Those Tapestry segments covered a range of lifestyles and socio-economic conditions:

- **Dorms to Diplomas** (22.7 percent response rate): With a median age of 21.5, these people live in neighborhoods with a mix of dorms and on-campus and off-campus housing that caters to young renters.

- **City Lights** (31.3 percent response rate): This group earns above-average incomes but lags the nation in net worth. Its median age is 38.8.

- **Young and Restless** (41.5 percent response rate): This highly mobile group with a median age of just under 30 is populated with people beginning careers and frequently changing addresses.

- **Modest Income Homes** (44.8 percent response rate): The labor force participation rate for this group is just 50 percent, with an income of less than half the US median. Most households rely heavily on public transportation.

- **Metro Fusion** (45.6 percent response rate): Single-parent and single-person households account for more than half of this group, with a median age of 28.8 and median household income of $33,000.

- **City Commons** (46.5 percent response rate): Nearly one-quarter of people in this group receive public assistance or Social Security benefits. They typically live in large cities and rent apartments in mid-rise buildings.

Once Census Bureau staff correlated nonresponders to the segment groups, they could perform deeper GIS analysis to find outreach opportunities, develop messaging, and tailor delivery.

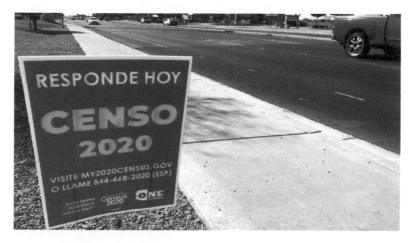

The message *Respond Today*, along with a website address and telephone number for the Census Bureau, went out in many languages, including Spanish on this sign in Phoenix, Arizona.

Marketing through smarter outreach

With insights gleaned from each segment profile, the bureau customized outreach for audiences deemed hard to find during the 2020 Census.

The Census Bureau met regularly with VMLY&R, the agency that secured the Integrated Communications Contract for the 2020 census campaign, to review where segments were under- or overreporting self-response, Bates said. "We then drew on mitigation plans to get self-response rates to where we wanted them to be."

Deeper knowledge of lifestyle segmentation groups helped Census Bureau staff detect patterns in how people respond to marketing. Direct mail, including flyers and cards with the web address of the online census form, prompted most of the web traffic during the Savannah test. Two segments, City Commons and Modest Income Homes, were the least likely to select the web for submitting their responses, averaging 54 percent. In contrast, the Young and Restless segment was about average, with 70 percent choosing the web

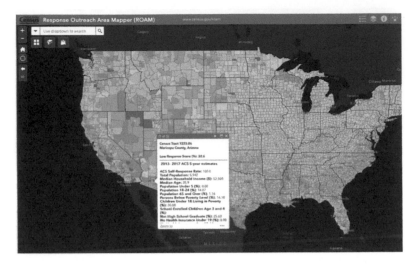

The Response Outreach Area Mapper (ROAM) application was developed to identify hard-to-survey areas and show socioeconomic and demographic profiles of these areas. Clicking any of the census tracts opens a pop-up with information about demographics, economic factors, and so on.

as the mode of response. Dorms to Diplomas, which had the lowest participation rate, had a relatively high web response rate of 77 percent—in line with attitudinal characteristics of the younger, tech-savvy segment.

The Census count corresponded to a time of heavy political advertising and the emergence of the pandemic with its public health and economic fallout. With lessons learned from the Savannah test, the Census Bureau responded quickly to market dynamics and increased its paid media investment.

Census Bureau workers used digital marketing to reach more people at higher frequency than was possible in 2010. A heavier digital imprint boosted participation among low-responding segments through search-engine-based digital ads and Facebook posts. In the earlier Savannah test, seniors responded at the highest rate to search engine ads (more than 80 percent), and singles responded the most to Facebook ads (more than 30 percent). These tendencies helped guide targeted ads in the 2020 Census.

"Some of the segments are really small, such as Student and Military Communities that make up just 2 percent of the US population," Bates said. "But knowing where those communities are helps us target their interests."

A metrics-driven marketing strategy helped improve 2020 Census response, even under the year's extraordinary circumstances. (The Census Bureau reported a self-response rate of 67 percent for the 2020 count, compared with 66.5 percent in 2010.) The Census Bureau's digital transformation included the application of GIS to gain location intelligence on population segments with typically low response rates. This transformation empowered staff to craft outreach based on lifestyle segmentation data. Ultimately, this updated approach supported a successful 2020 Census count even during a pandemic.

A version of this story by Karisa Schroeder originally appeared as "Census Bureau Taps Location Intelligence to Boost Response Rates" on the *Esri Blog* on February 11, 2021.

WELCOME

WE ARE

OPEN

PLEASE COME IN

PART 5

RECOVERY AND RESILIENCE

PERHAPS ABOVE ALL ELSE, THE PANDEMIC HAS TAUGHT US that the road to recovery is demanding, confounding, and tiring. The path to a new normal requires consideration of various trade-offs. Ideally, we want to prioritize health above all other considerations; realistically, we can't avoid every viral threat or health risk that comes our way. Given the social and economic determinants of health, we know that staying healthy involves a combination of many contextual factors and conditions. A person who loses their job during pandemic shutdowns, for example, may consequently lose their health insurance coverage. Perhaps their next opportunity is a customer service position that requires frequent contact with the general public, thus raising the risk of exposure. The exigencies of health require that we also recognize the interconnectedness of our world.

As we address recovery and resilience, we'll see how GIS technology can support the balance between economic sustainability and health security. That balance begins with a framework for decision-making. It starts with evaluating economic and health trends so we can weigh both measures in our decision-making. As we learned in part 2, recovery and resilience require a methodology to assess community and organizational needs and vulnerabilities. The goal is to support the near-term needs of healing and the long-term essentials that boost strength, resilience, and flex-ibility for whatever comes next. As initiatives are implemented, we must develop metrics to monitor their progress. In that context, GIS supports the communication of recovery and resilience programs in transparent, engaging, and galvanizing ways.

In this section, spatial statisticians Lauren Scott Griffin and Kevin Butler share explicit directions on evaluating a community's readiness for relaxing stay-at-home orders. The lessons they share go well beyond a single analytic workflow, serving as a best-practices guide to systematic investigation: determine key objectives, ask the right questions, assemble data resources, perform the analysis, and interpret results.

As many businesses have reopened their workplaces, consider-ations about what it means to achieve organizational recovery and resilience have come to the fore. How can a business pivot and adapt in response to a global crisis? Having the best information is par-amount. Modern technologies access information faster and more easily than ever before. Since the late 1990s, our embedded, nearly ubiquitous connectivity has drawn us into what some are calling a fourth industrial revolution. The pandemic hastened the revolu-tion's blurring of boundaries between physical and digital worlds. Many people survived economically because they could do their jobs remotely. As the pandemic evolved, many companies transitioned to permanent remote work, while others implemented hybrid sys-tems. For everyone returning to a workplace, ensuring their safety and health is of utmost importance.

In this section, you'll learn about the steps to reopen work-places in indoor environments with physical distancing. Accommo-dating new work patterns such as hoteling (reserving an available workspace ahead of time) and hot desking (choosing a workspace after arriving to work) requires a paradigm shift for managers and employees and a new way to envision the physical workspace. Indoor GIS helps organizations oversee seat assignments, monitor employees in buildings, support public health contact tracing efforts, and more. GIS can promote the same kind of situational awareness and common operating picture described in part 1 for brick and mortar spaces. These stories explain how organizations can allocate office space to highest advantage and identify cleaning and maintenance needs with streamlined efficiency. The goal is to keep businesses and people safe and productive.

Earlier, we examined the supply chain from the perspective of Direct Relief, a nonprofit organization that moves medical supplies to places in need, usually during disasters. The stories in this section view the supply chain from the business perspective. How does a business react to changes in the availability of essential goods? Is the current supply chain geographically diverse enough to mitigate an emergency in another part of the chain? Can the business modify supply orders to a *just-in-time* system over a *just-in-case* system? You'll see that whether supplies are health oriented or business oriented, the geography of decision-making remains critical.

This section also explores how Pennsylvania counties used location-based tools to assess economic fallout from the pandemic. Survey123 and ArcGIS Hub play central roles in this endeavor, facilitating quick data capture, collaboration among neighboring jurisdictions, and communication among those who need to know. Part 5 of this book concludes with a discussion between mapping experts about practical ways to create a common operating picture of an organization's facilities and ensure a new level of safety in the workplace.

Resilience is not a given—it is built through time, experiences, hardship, and careful planning. From one community to another and from one organization to the next, the path to building resilience is unique. Each place engenders its own characteristics, assets, and flaws. Each seesaw or balance scale will weigh its own local metrics and outcomes. And each fulcrum must be adjusted in different directions over different schedules to achieve or maintain balance. It's complicated. But GIS can help unravel that complexity by helping to reduce impacts to vulnerable communities and organizations, support their recovery needs, and build a foundation for a better future.

FIVE SPATIAL APPROACHES TO SAFELY REOPENING

Esri

AS COMMUNITIES HAVE REOPENED AFTER COVID-19 closures, leaders at all levels of government and business have relied on geospatial technology to help monitor and safeguard public health. Building on these efforts, they have also used GIS capabilities to guide safe reopening strategies.

Here are five recommended approaches to reopening with GIS:

1. Map the trends

Of special concern is the ability to stay vigilant and quell future waves of COVID-19 cases. The well-documented flu pandemic of 1918–1919 was deadliest during its second wave of infections. Today, we are far more aware and connected, with maps that show current, time-enabled information for monitoring infection trends daily.

Maps and dashboards allow us to quickly see many key aspects of the COVID-19 crisis. They show us whether cases are spreading and spiking and help us determine whether the outbreak is controlled. They help identify local hot spots to provide focused services for people in need. And, as the crisis has evolved, many jurisdictions developed more granular views of the spread of cases, with dashboards showing cases by postal code.

Epidemiologists and local health authorities appreciate the capability of spatial analytics and maps to deliver a data-driven response. They use models for projections of case increases, mapped against scenarios with differing levels of social distancing compliance, and use that insight to plan increased hospital capacity as surges occur. Mapping the trends provides a data-driven method for boosting

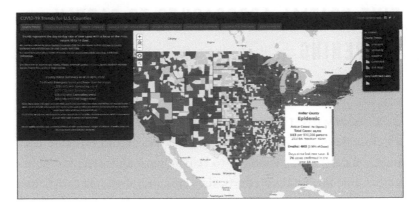

Mapping the day-to-day rate of new cases at the county level provides
an important input to understand areas where COVID-19 is emergent,
spreading, or controlled. Clicking a county provides a pop-up with detailed
information on active cases, total cases, case rate, deaths, and more.

response measures, staying the course, and pivoting toward recovery efforts.

2. Map for community resilience

The COVID-19 pandemic brought about many changes in the ways
we live our public lives. It highlighted the importance of understanding
human interactions, partly because of the relationship between
proximity and viral spread. Consequently, information about where
people are and how they are interacting is essential to the ongoing
safety, security, and well-being of our communities.

To maintain and increase community resilience, leaders can use
the geospatial toolset to monitor how people interact and move and
then make data-driven decisions to support population needs and
safety for each location.

The stories in part 1 revolved around the value and use of situational
awareness. Through GIS-enabled location analytics, we can
detect and visualize patterns in real time, spot anomalies, and gain

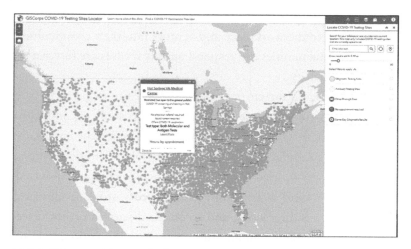

URISA (Urban and Regional Information Systems Association) GISCorps volunteers created a national COVID-19 testing site locator map where visitors can find and submit sites where testing services are available.

insights. That section of the book further discussed how contact tracing can help leaders quell the spread of disease by understanding linkages beyond cases and contacts to include the places people have visited—a new effort called community contact tracing. These foundational efforts also underpin interventions for community resilience by providing evidence for the effectiveness of measures to ensure health security while reopening.

As people take part in social and cultural activities again, GIS tools can assist in the planning and managing of physical distancing to prevent new transmission chains of the virus. If cases begin to increase again, GIS can help monitor human mobility data and look for areas of concern among anonymized data points from mobile devices.

By monitoring demand for government services by location, leaders can prioritize areas where more support may be needed. Leaders also need to regularly monitor and assess health system capacity as people return to the workplace and venture into their communities. In this way, communities can respond quickly if cases are forecast to overwhelm capacity.

GIS map-based directories offer a simple, intuitive way to connect residents to government services, health services, and businesses—and these resource locators have never been more important. Municipalities around the world, such as Cobb County, Georgia, described in part 4, used a similar approach to create map-based directories for food distribution sites, grocery store inventories, essential business directories, and so on. As discussed earlier, if we are to ensure resilient communities, we must be intentional about analyzing service delivery, not only to meet demand but to uncover disparities and provide equitable care and services for everyone.

3. Map for organizational resilience

COVID-19 disruptions hit businesses particularly hard. GIS provides business leaders with operational awareness to help stabilize and reestablish their trade after cases are controlled. Businesses with many physical locations use GIS to monitor the status of their facilities and retail outlets. They use GIS dashboards to review individual performance, compile and react to differing infection rates and regulations in all locations, and make strategic reopening plans. GIS is also used to monitor complex global supply chains, many of which have been disrupted by global factory closures.

Many businesses use online maps to assess and display measures of staff safety and wellness for employees deemed essential for on-site work and those working from home or in the field. Map-based awareness allows businesses to visualize personnel resources and to efficiently relocate staff based on current needs and conditions.

As business leaders plan and assess the return of their workforces to office locations, indoor mapping can address the use of space and

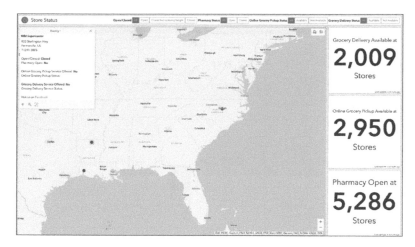

Walmart created a national store status locator map to display which stores were open and what services were available for grocery and pharmacy supplies.

support social distancing. An indoor view (described later in this section) helps companies prepare and respond should an employee become infected—giving managers the information they need to warn and quarantine possible contacts. A real-time map of indoor spaces allows a business to monitor sanitization operations and react to safety concerns.

4. Map the impacts

Map-based applications and dashboards help leaders quickly assess the impacts of the COVID-19 crisis. Economic indicators such as unemployment levels, new business licenses, and tourism revenues can provide local context on economic strength and vulnerability. Leaders from business and government can then use the map-based data to understand the local issues to respond and plan.

As businesses and governments strive toward economic recovery, they must carefully monitor economic and health indicators to

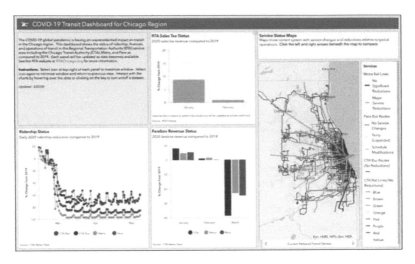

The Regional Transportation Authority uses a dashboard to display and monitor the unprecedented impact on ridership and revenue in the Chicago region.

maintain an appropriate balance. To do so, organizations can tap into available COVID-19 case data from local, state, and federal authorities to see changes in case levels and create alerts if locations face increasing risk. With location-based data, they can be strategic about when and where it is prudent to strengthen social distancing measures. On the flip side, when case data indicates decreasing infection rates, appropriate relaxing of controls can be considered to stimulate economic interests.

5. Communicate with maps

Although national policy certainly plays a role in how locations recover from the COVID-19 crisis, most actions take place locally. It is here that policies and resulting behaviors have the most immediate impact. Local governments and various businesses have created multiple map-based apps to address different facets of this crisis, and

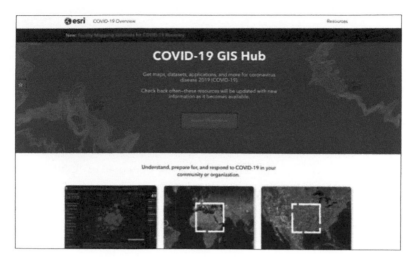

Esri's COVID-19 GIS Hub compiles maps, data, and applications directed at understanding and responding to COVID-19.

they use the community engagement tool, ArcGIS Hub, to organize and display this information, as described in part 4.

Esri used this same configurable tool to create the COVID-19 GIS Hub, which compiles resources and applications that support GIS users around the world as they understand, prepare, and respond. A combination of map-based communication tools—interactive web maps, dashboard apps, and ArcGIS StoryMaps stories—helps organizations rapidly relate constantly changing conditions.

Communities around the world have taken a data- and mapcentric approach to the first pandemic of the digital age. Never before have we seen such a global desire for real-time and near real-time information. Governments and businesses are also engaged—analyzing and conveying details that help constituents, residents, employees, and customers understand local impacts. Because ArcGIS is flexible, it allows people to tailor messaging and resources to their own circumstances.

As jurisdictions have worked to meet health benchmarks for reopening and economic health, map-based views will continue to help. Organizations at all scales will use GIS to map, measure, model, and monitor reopening iteratively across the waves of the COVID-19 crisis. A focused awareness of the power of geographic thinking is essential for keeping communities and businesses safe and healthy.

A version of this story by Este Geraghty originally appeared as "COVID-19: Five Spatial Approaches to Safely Reopen" on the *Esri Blog* on June 2, 2020.

EVALUATING READINESS FOR RELAXING STAY-AT-HOME MEASURES

Esri

DURING THE PANDEMIC, WE LEARNED THAT SOCIAL distancing and stay-at-home policies saved lives and helped flatten the COVID-19 curve. We also learned about the economic impacts of these policies, as millions of people across the United States filed for unemployment amid shuttered businesses and overwhelmed food banks. Governors faced mounting pressure to relax, modify, or lift the social distancing and stay-at-home policies imposed to keep people safe. Can GIS help governments find compromises and solutions? Yes.

This story outlines a data-driven approach for evaluating stay-at-home measures that could apply to this pandemic or the aftermath of any future pandemic. The approach is presented in three parts:

- A high-level overview of the proposed workflow

- An example of applying the workflow to objectives for California counties

- A step-by-step tutorial, with data and available in the resources for this book, allowing GIS analysts to practice the workflow before applying it to their own data (see the link to "Evaluate County Readiness for Relaxing Stay-at-Home Measures" at go.esri.com/lfc-resources)

Overview

Evaluating stay-at-home orders—in response to this pandemic or to a new one—requires starting at the beginning. What are your objectives and goals? How might they be measured? No doubt you want to protect people, monitor policy impacts, foster equity, respond to consequences, and promote good health and a strong economy.

1. Engage with stakeholders, particularly those in communities most strongly impacted, as you create a list of your key objectives.

2. Identify data sources and data variables available to track impacts and progress.

3. Standardize, weigh, and sum each data variable to create a score reflecting readiness for modified stay-at-home policies.

4. Map the scores to identify where to begin and how to proceed.

5. Evaluate the impacts.

6. As difficult as it is, you must answer the hardest questions:

   - What are the threshold values for COVID-19 deaths and hospitalizations that would trigger reinstating stay-at-home orders?

   - What are the acceptable limits for job and business losses that would lead to more relaxed stay-at-home policies?

Example: California

Governor Gavin Newsom outlined these objectives for California:

1. The ability to monitor and protect communities through testing, contact tracing, isolating, and supporting those who are positive or exposed

2. The ability to prevent infection in people who are at risk to develop severe symptoms of COVID-19

3. The ability of hospitals and health systems to handle surges

4. The ability to develop therapeutics to meet demands

5. The ability for businesses, schools, and childcare facilities to support physical distancing

6. The ability to determine when to reinstitute specific measures such as the stay-at-home orders, if necessary

Before modifying stay-at-home measures, leaders must reach out to communities facing the highest risk:

- Health care and other frontline workers

- Communal facilities such as nursing homes, military barracks, and jails

- Black and Hispanic communities to ensure equitable access to testing, treatment, and other vital resources

- School staff working in classrooms and cafeterias

- Small businesses, especially those providing services requiring face-to-face contact with clients

A successful outcome requires understanding the daily challenges of those hardest hit by COVID-19 and its economic consequences. A data-driven analysis converts objectives into metrics for use in assessing, monitoring, and tracking impacts and efficacy. California's objectives, for example, might convert into the next list of potential data variables. The variables in **bold** are for demonstration purposes in the tutorial available in the online resources for this book.

Monitor (objective 1):

- Number of tests performed, number of people active with the virus, **confirmed cases, deaths,** new cases, new deaths, and percentage of the population who have recovered or have tested positive for antibodies

- Access to testing (promoting equity based on need)

Protect (objective 1):

- Trained staff available to perform contact tracing or percentage of the population participating in automated contact tracing

- Ratio of **public health staff to total population**

- Number of people with employer-covered job protection and paid sick leave

- Availability of economic and other support services for families with sick individuals

- A measure of the impact and effectiveness of economic stimulus programs

Prevent (objective 2):

- Availability or inventory of PPE

- A measure of effectiveness of programs to prevent and contain infections across health care facilities, such as **nursing homes,** hospitals, jails, and shelters

- The number of people in the highest risk categories (older people, **Black and Hispanic populations**, those suffering from chronic illnesses and other underlying health conditions, families living in poverty, the unemployed, people experiencing homelessness, multigenerational households, group housing residents, and so on)

- A measure of the progress made in sanitation and deep-cleaning efforts

Respond (objective 3):

- Necessary hospital resources: health care professionals, **staffed beds, ICU beds**, ventilators, respirators, pharmaceuticals, training

- Epidemiological model predictions for COVID-19 surges and capacity requirements

Treat (objective 4):

- Percentage of population with **health insurance coverage**

- Availability of effective antivirals and other therapeutics

- Availability of a vaccine

Comply (objective 5):

- **Measures of social and spatial interaction**

- Percentage of employers implementing prevention and containment measures (practicing social distancing; requiring employees to be vaccinated and get tested, wear masks, and take temperatures; allowing employees to work from home, and so on)

- Percentage of schools and other childcare facilities implementing protective strategies (practicing social distancing, regular handwashing, vaccination, staggering classes, remote education opportunities, and so on)

- Percentage of families with access to computers and broadband

- Percentage of population working away from home

- Percentage of the population working in essential jobs (unable to stay home)

Evaluate (objective 6):

- The number of **new cases and new deaths**

- **Changes in social distancing and spatial interaction**

- Changes in unemployment

- Measures of economic prosperity

You won't have access to every piece of data listed, and you will likely want to include other variables in your analyses. The variables for California's objectives focus on health, safety, and protection. Other states might want to include additional economic variables (such as employment data for the industries and occupations most critical to the economy). Move forward with what you have, making improvements as additional data becomes available.

Standardize, weigh, and sum each variable

For some of the collected variables, high values are better (available hospital beds and social distancing scores, for example). For other variables, low values are better (new confirmed cases and health facility citations). In addition, the variables you collect may have different units of measurement (counts, percentages, dollars, and so on). By standardizing the variables, you address both issues: you reclassify the data so all values range from 0.0 to 1.0, and you ensure consistency so low values always reflect the best or most desired situations and high values always reflect the worst scenarios. Although standardizing the variables gives them an equal scale and direction, it does not deal with differences in variable importance. For this part of the analysis, you'll assign a weight to each variable. You may decide, for example, to assign weights between 1 and 5. The least important variables would then be assigned weight values at or near 1, and the most important variables would be assigned weight values at or near 5. To get a single score for each county, you'll sum the standardized, weighted values.

Map the scores

Mapping the final scores would show which counties were most prepared for relaxing stay-at-home measures. After relaxing or lifting some of the restrictions, you could evaluate the impacts by tracking the number of new COVID-19 cases, new deaths, and changes in social distancing. You could also track unemployment and other economic indicators. Monitoring this data could help determine whether authorities need to reinstate, maintain, or further relax stay-at-home measures.

A version of this story by Lauren Scott Griffin and Kevin Butler originally appeared as "Evaluate County Readiness for Relaxing Stay-at-Home Measures" on the *ArcGIS Blog* on May 1, 2020.

ASSESSING ECONOMIC FALLOUT WITH SHARED MAPS

Montgomery, Bucks, Chester, and Delaware Counties, and the city and county of Philadelphia, Pennsylvania

W HEN THE COVID-19 PANDEMIC REACHED PENNSYLVANIA in early 2020, it hit Montgomery County first. By March 12, 2020, these northern Philadelphia suburbs accounted for 13 of the commonwealth's first 22 reported cases.

In the weeks leading up to the local coronavirus outbreak, businesses throughout the Philadelphia metro area had braced for its impact. More than 20 local organizations—comprising experts in economic development, small business management, tourism, destination marketing, international business, the technology sector, and venture capital—had already traded notes on strategies to support the business community.

Economic development officials in several counties and municipalities had also begun to conduct informal surveys of local business owners to gauge how the outbreak had affected them so far, what they feared would happen next, and what kind of assistance they would need.

Early in the pandemic, several officials floated the idea of collaborating on survey efforts. Montgomery County took the lead, organizing a centralized survey of businesses that extended to the neighboring counties of Bucks, Chester, and Delaware, and the city and county of Philadelphia. Taken together, the survey would add up to a detailed economic picture of a swath of the Delaware Valley.

"Economies do not stop at community or county borders," said David Zellers, Montgomery County's director of commerce. "We need to work together as a regional team to flip the switch when economy is ready to start again."

The first round of surveys went out on Friday, March 13, 2020. That first weekend, 440 surveys were returned. By the end of the month, the effort had yielded useful data from more than 1,000 businesses and companies.

Understanding economic fallout in different sectors across different areas

The surveys were a way for officials like Zellers to chart how COVID-19 had affected businesses across various sizes and sectors.

Although the region itself is economically and demographically interdependent, there are distinct ways in which certain types of businesses felt the crunch. Location intelligence is a vital aspect of the analysis, helping answer important questions that affect strategies:

- In a time of social distancing, will the density of Philadelphia serve as a help or a hindrance?

- In the suburbs and exurbs, will a declining population in office parks and campuses have a ripple effect for nearby support businesses?

- As government aid flows into the region, will certain areas see more of it than others?

To help answer these questions—and, just as importantly, to visualize answers—a GIS will retain relevant data. Interactive GIS maps can provide an intuitive way to see how businesses in different areas handle the difficult task of rebuilding. GIS dashboards can bring in other types of datasets, such as unemployment statistics and revenue from tourism.

"I think as we gather more results and we look beyond the immediate public health situation, geospatial analysis is going to be very important," Zellers said in 2020. "We will start understanding where the impacts have been and the magnitude of those impacts across sectors and across communities."

A connection to the past, a bridge to the future

There is a poignant historical aspect to this effort to understand the effect of COVID-19 on the Philadelphia area. During the massive Spanish flu pandemic of 1918–1919 that killed at least 50 million people worldwide, Philadelphia was one of the hardest-hit American cities. Nearly one of four residents of the city contracted the disease and more than 16,000 died. During the COVID-19 pandemic, some 5,085 residents had died as of mid-April 2022.

In this context, the economic fallout survey is an important building block for the region's future. The area is a central hub for such industries as finance, advanced manufacturing, pharmaceuticals, life sciences, and logistics.

Zellers sees the survey as a longitudinal study that documents the rebuilding of the area's economy over an extended period. In the coming months—and even years—the study will help officials and researchers learn about more than just the Delaware Valley economy. It will also help them understand the rebuilding of all the world's advanced economies.

Zellers views GIS as key to this understanding for its ability to give numbers and statistics a real-world context. "The analytical piece of this is so important—and being able to visualize all of this makes a huge difference," he said.

Officials believe the project will serve as a model for the collaborative approach essential for rebuilding local economies.

"Recovery is not a siloed process," Zellers explained. "We want our communities to know, and we want our elected leaders to know, that we're working together on this. We're united, not just in collecting data but also in the strategies we want to promote to help every person here move past what's happening right now and have a stronger region in the future."

Mapping the economy of the Delaware Valley

The effort to survey and map the effect of the COVID-19 outbreak on five Philadelphia-area counties, using ArcGIS Survey123 to gather responses, was just the beginning. As completed surveys returned, officials began to focus on building out the economic fallout map.

"So far [April 2020], we've mainly done some heat mapping to understand where the surveys are coming from," said David Long, GIS manager for Montgomery County. "For now, that's our main task."

In time, Long predicts the economic fallout map will help the counties advocate for businesses and direct relief efforts. "If the county applies for relief funds, our Commerce Department can use this data to target certain industries that seem to be hit hardest, based on the survey and the map," Long said.

A version of this story by Richard Leadbeater originally appeared as "COVID-19: Pennsylvania Counties Assess Economic Fallout with Shared Maps" on the *Esri Blog* on April 8, 2020.

BALANCING RESPONSE AND RECOVERY

Esri

F OR MOST EVERYONE IN THE WORLD, THE COVID-19 CRISIS came as a bolt from the blue. And although there have been disruptions in global supply chains before (during world wars and tsunamis, for instance), COVID-19 has taken a heavy economic toll on global producers, distributors, logistics providers, retailers, and consumers.

Understandably, companies and organizations of every type focused initially on mitigating the medical and public health dimensions of the crisis, but with time it was clear that the planning must also include strategies to stem the economic fallout, which has been considerable.

The outbreak plunged the global economy into recession almost overnight. The world's GDP dropped over 3 percent for 2020, according to the IHS Markit Economics & Country Risk study. We saw historic levels of job losses. While reopening the economy is not an economic cure-all, agile companies have used GIS to minimize their own economic fallout. They shifted supply chains from commercial toward consumer markets and marshaled resources in locations where people, products, and services were needed most.

Business leaders focused on three phases of business activity: protect, stabilize, and reestablish. In each phase, they have used information hubs that feature location intelligence to guide decisions. These hubs provide different datasets to different users, giving customers, employees, and partners needed data. Stakeholders can use insights from the data to adjust plans and processes to fit current conditions.

A response based on good data, effective communication

The first step was to protect against the immediate health threats to employees and operations. Next, companies assessed and stabilized

available resources to meet shifting demands. After that, execut
planned for the longer term, reestablishing their business whe.
and when possible, with an eye toward recovery. So what does it
look like to resume a normal business cadence in the context of a
pandemic?

It begins with location data and communication. With help from
business information hubs, companies can share workforce and operations data internally and externally. Communicating with employees is especially important for workforce health—knowing who is
well enough to come to work at essential businesses, for example.
In many cases, employees submit this information through mobile
devices. GIS technology automatically contextualizes that data on
smart maps for real-time sharing across the organization. This same
technology serves as the platform for business information hubs.

Location information has been a communications driver during
this lingering pandemic, helping executives visualize the geographic
landscape of their workforces in the context of current business
activities. Other companies augment those smart maps with data
on operations—for example, where customers are using products
and services, and how those habits may have changed. This capability helps executives with the task of resourcing to meet consumer
demands.

A glimpse at recovery

Grocery chains and food services addressed surging local demand
during the pandemic by providing a safe environment for customers and employees. They began curbside delivery, installed plexiglass
barriers, implemented social distancing, limited capacity, set special
hours for seniors, and offered hazard pay, among many examples.
Other kinds of business have also used location intelligence to adjust
their operations.

Consider the hypothetical scenario of a multistate company that anufactures sanitizing products and provides on-site cleaning services to facilities. Its response to the COVID-19 situation might begin with a basic awareness of its employees' locations and health status. Employees provide this information by completing a daily survey on their mobile phones. That data flows into the information hub and gives company leaders a reliable view of workforce well-being. The hub also delivers helpful information to employees, including near real-time maps of local resources such as health care facilities and businesses that remain open.

Meanwhile, the company's operations managers broaden their focus to the challenge of resourcing. They start by examining which organizations still operate in their customer base. Hospitals and medical offices count as essential businesses that need sanitizing products and cleaning services, likely in greater quantities than usual. In contrast, the company's business serving restaurants and educational institutions has essentially dried up. Executives must reallocate resources to focus on the surge in health care—and flatten the business disruption.

The company's GIS team creates a smart map—an interactive map that allows data exploration—with several overlapping layers of information to help managers make resourcing decisions. One layer shows the location of high-demand customer sites. Another reveals product availability at each regional distribution center, and a third layer shows where personnel can deliver on-site cleaning services. Behind the scenes, the data is being collected and organized by the information hub, creating a central source of insight for fast decisions to keep pace with operational challenges.

While the company's health care customers still need support, the education sector presumably will not need hand sanitizer and cleaning services as long as schools remain closed. Office buildings fall somewhere in between, but as businesses and schools reopen, the need for hand sanitizer and cleaning services will increase, and thes services will become more important than before. Accordingly, the company can shift personnel as much as possible to the geographic areas where essential services and supplies are needed.

Executives must shape plans for recovery in the real world too. Companies will continue to adjust services, products, workforce, facilities, and distribution channels as their markets evolve along with the pandemic. Geographic insights will inform everything from high-level business survival strategy to granular decisions, such as identifying regions where truck drivers still need to wear masks during product deliveries.

A challenge for every industry

In every pocket of the economy, location data supports companies as they move toward recovery in a way that makes sense for each organization. Executives worldwide are trying to understand demand in specific locations and shift employees and resources accordingly. Organizations with proactive GIS leadership can see all relevant information in a single location—an information hub that tracks how the business is running, and where it needs to adjust.

Few if any in government or business seem to have anticipated the full impact of COVID-19. But as important progress is made on the public health front, businesses can implement strategies to recover economically. As they do, leadership must be nimble and responsive to market indicators, including government guidelines, public sentiment, and customer needs. Through location intelligence, they can gauge the tenor of each market—even each neighborhood—and time business recovery to an area's readiness to reopen.

A version of this story by Cindy Elliott originally appeared as "COVID-19: Balancing Response and Recovery" in WhereNext on April 28, 2020.

HOW TO REOPEN THE WORKPLACE DURING COVID-19

Esri

THE COVID-19 PANDEMIC HAS CHANGED THE RULES OF human interaction, and not just in the short term. To respond, business and organizational leaders must establish a new definition of workplace safety for their facilities.

In this story, Esri's Brian Cross talks to indoor mapping experts Will Isley and Beau Ryck about the conversations they're having with business leaders, what it means to establish a common operating picture of an organization's facilities, and how to create a new level of safety in the workplace.

Brian Cross: We've explored the trend of indoor mapping in the past, and that topic is quickly gaining attention as business leaders contemplate new patterns of work and challenges to safety and health in the workplace.

To put this in perspective, I thought we could start by discussing what workplace challenges executives were solving with indoor maps before COVID-19.

Beau Ryck: The main challenge has been developing a system of record that organizes building and floor plan data. Employers use this to improve workplace experiences for employees and visitors—through wayfinding and room-booking applications, for example. They also use the data to manage maintenance more efficiently. Indoor maps create a common operating picture that allows them to manage buildings and equipment as assets.

Cross: Now you're both helping companies address new priorities as they respond to COVID-19. We'll explore those in a minute, but I'm curious whether you see this pandemic having long-term effects on the workplace.

Will Isley: I think COVID-19 will change the workplace in ing ways—similar to the way September 11 changed security pra tices in the airline industry. Safety has always been a basic premise of the workplace, but you might say it lived in the background. Now it's at the top of every executive's agenda and will be for the foreseeable future. Companies have to protect their employees, because if workers are not safe, operations cannot continue.

Ryck: I agree. Safety challenges in the workplace won't go away once the COVID-19 threat fades. Natural and human-made disasters will continue to occur, and executives will need situational awareness of their facilities to manage those events. I think the pandemic will drive businesses toward better systems for dealing with hazards and disaster planning. Longer term, as business leaders grow more comfortable with a remote workforce and flexible working schedules, some might even reevaluate their real estate holdings and shed leases. It's really interesting to see how mapping technology is helping guide these decisions.

Navigating a new world of work

Cross: In the COVID-19 world, what are some emerging uses for indoor mapping?

Isley: Indoor maps are being used in three aspects of the COVID-19 pandemic. The first is direct response. This mostly involves frontline locations like hospitals, shelters, pop-up facilities, and campuses that are providing emergency services and health care. They need to understand how to adapt their indoor space to accommodate physical distancing, help people find the resources they need, understand and address facility issues, define new health and safety procedures, and more.

The second use for indoor mapping involves managing indoor environments when employees return to work. Companies need to map out seat assignments and safety procedures and understand

...o's in the office, who's not. They also need to know where maintenance has been performed and how physical systems are operating.

The third is advanced analysis of the indoor environment.
For example, companies are preparing response plans in case an
employee contracts the virus. They're looking to create a common
operating picture—a real-time map—of the workplace. That's a new
level of indoor awareness for most companies.

How executives are rethinking indoor space

Cross: I imagine a lot of the executives you work with are focused on
adjusting physical layouts and procedures when they begin to reopen
offices. What does that involve?

Ryck: Before the COVID-19 outbreak, companies were focused
on maximizing space usage, since property is usually the second-big-
gest expense on their books. In some cases, they did this through
space-sharing practices such as hoteling (reserving a workspace
ahead of time) and hot desking (choosing an open workspace
after arriving). Some of those practices will survive this pandemic
and perhaps even thrive—especially since many employees will
work remotely part of the time. But much more governance will be
involved. Employees won't be able to show up at the office and grab
an available desk.

Hoteling, for instance, is a managed process—it can be run on
interactive maps that account for social distancing. Employees can
reserve space on the map, managers can approve the assignments,
and the system will alert maintenance staff when shared spaces need
to be sanitized.

We also see planners using space analysis to find choke points in
their facilities and reduce the possibility of congestion. They're using
indoor maps to adjust the space and ensure physical distancing.

Data points toward phased openings

Cross: I imagine executives with facilities in multiple states might find it difficult to gauge the readiness of each property. How will they decide when and how to open facilities?

Isley: The business leaders we've talked to are doing location analysis. They know that the COVID-19 reality in New Jersey, for instance, is very different from that in Idaho. Even within a state, infection rates and risk levels vary substantially by location.

Executives know how important good data is to good decisions, so they're using technology like GIS for analysis. For example, they might use GIS to analyze data on COVID-19 trends, including statistics such as the number of days since a county's last reported COVID-19 case and the status of its infection rate, from spreading to end stage. That gives decision-makers the location intelligence they need to make plans specific to each facility.

Ryck: This is where traditional GIS and indoor GIS intersect. Once executives gauge the readiness of each facility based on state and local data, they'll map out new procedures within each facility.

Cross: How will they deal with the variations across locations—how will that process play out?

Isley: We expect many companies to create a tiered reopening system. A facility at tier two, for example, might enforce certain rules: open space seating is prohibited, no more than 40 percent of the workforce can be in the workplace, and social distancing is managed very strictly. For a facility at tier four, that might mean 75 percent of the workforce is back in the office, visitors are allowed with special permission, and common spaces are open but with limited seating in lunch areas.

Employers will design and manage those scenarios on smart maps. When local and county-level laws and data indicate that a facility can move to the next level of openness, a manager can click on the relevant tier in GIS, and the indoor map will display the game plan for that tier—for managers and employees.

Responding to instances of COVID-19 infection among employees

Cross: Despite their best efforts to protect employees, companies could still face a situation where an employee contracts COVID-19. How will organizations deal with that?

Ryck: The White House issued guidelines stating that employers should be prepared to implement contact tracing if an employee tests positive for COVID-19. The guidelines are not specific about how that should happen, so companies are looking for best practices.

Some companies are using location technology on mobile devices to allow staff to self-report. If I'm working from home for the day, I check in on the app, report where I'm working, and note if I have any COVID-19 symptoms. Managers see a map of who is in the office and who is off-site, and what everyone's status is.

This mapping capability supports basic contact tracing because employee check-ins are saved for a certain period—say, three weeks. If an employee reports symptoms, a manager can essentially rewind the map over the past two weeks and see which colleagues that employee may have come into contact with.

We're working with large organizations in public and private sectors that are doing this for thousands of employees.

Isley: In certain high-risk work environments, companies will want to do more rigorous contact tracing. They will use a combination of mobile devices and indoor positioning technologies like Wi-Fi access points or Bluetooth beacons to understand where employees are as they move through facilities. Apple, Google, and other tech companies are providing SDKs (software development kits) for proximity detection, too. If someone tests positive for the virus, rithms in GIS technology can help managers figure out who that son came into contact with.

Restarting operations

Cross: So far, we've focused on employee activity, but what about the physical operations of offices and workplaces?

Ryck: If facilities have been largely unoccupied or running at minimal capacity for some time, organizations will want to ensure that mechanical systems are functioning safely as operations resume. Historically, maintenance involved a lot of paper-based work orders and physical handoffs. The trend of using digital maps to integrate with work-order systems—to manage everything from sanitizing common areas to changing air filters—will accelerate. That minimizes in-person contact and helps with social distancing.

The common operating picture moves indoors

Cross: What I'm hearing across this conversation is that leaders are interested in creating a common operating picture of the workplace. They need to see the workplace in ways they never have before. They need to know how many offices are occupied, where staff are congregating, and which areas need cleaning. Indoor maps are creating that operating picture for managers and executives.

Isley: And for employees, too. Because as space plans change, employees will need to adapt. Some will end up in different office locations, and all will have new procedures to follow. Having an indoor map available on their computers or their phones will give them the information they need—everything from which areas are off-limits and where hand sanitizer stations are to the best way to navigate to a conference room or café.

That map will be their common operating picture, and it will

ate as facilities graduate to fewer restrictions, based on local con-
tions. This level of awareness will be key to keeping employees safe
in a new environment—and helping them and the businesses they
represent remain as productive as possible.

A version of this story by Chris Chiappinelli originally appeared as "Think
Tank: How to Reopen the Workplace during COVID-19" in *WhereNext* on
May 12, 2020.

COVID-19: OUR LESSONS LEARNED

CAPTURING THE LESSONS LEARNED DURING AND immediately after an emergency response or health crisis is key to the overall success of the public health preparedness profession. This proactive step puts software, data, expertise, and working relationships in place before the next crisis. In this way, communities are not forced to cobble together insights in the midst of a crisis, when everyone is struggling to address the massive demand on public health care.

The effects of the pandemic cascaded through society in ways far beyond the tragic loss of life and immeasurable trauma in its wake. We have learned that a complex public health emergency such as COVID-19 can touch on nearly every aspect of life, from transportation and education to economic development and public policy. For example, statewide shelter-in-place orders designed to save lives caused millions of people to lose their jobs and incomes. At the same time, school closures to protect children and educators interrupted the free breakfast and lunch programs many families rely on. Food supply chains were disrupted as restaurants closed or limited services and hours while consumer demand for groceries increased. This dislocation for suppliers and increased demand on grocery stores was exacerbated because they had come to rely on constant shipments and rapid restocking of goods. Widespread panic buying and hoarding compounded these logistics problems, leading to empty store shelves. So, although health agencies might lead the pandemic esponse, they also consider the scope of effects as they work closely with myriad governmental departments, nonprofit organizations, community businesses, and elected officials to plan, coordinate, and communicate response efforts.

Public health professionals will continue to evolve their use of technology to adapt preparedness, response, and recovery efforts after the COVID-19 pandemic. But response efforts during the pandemic presented an initial road map of core competencies required to improve an organization's response capacity and recommend programs, plans, policies, laws, and workforce development. The new terms and workflows can be incorporated into preparedness plans for a global crisis such as a pandemic, a large-scale emergency such as a hurricane, or a smaller-scale event such as a localized heat wave.

Learning from the past

Past emergencies have shown us how to extend the public health preparedness network to improve the exchange of information and outcomes to impacted areas.

- The 1994 Northridge earthquake in California demonstrated the need to coordinate with cellular carriers to use data to locate people.

- The Oklahoma City bombing in 1995 introduced 3D modeling.

- Hurricane Katrina in 2005 introduced improved coordination of displaced communities and volunteer efforts.

- The Deepwater Horizon oil spill in 2010 showed the need to protect tourism after an emergency.

Minimum data requirements shift depending on whether the in...
is the result of weather, fire, terrorism, or disease. The list of ...
resources a public health department collects for preparedness actr
ities becomes more comprehensive as the agency responds to a range
and frequency of events.

- The September 11, 2001, terrorist attacks showed how up-to-
  date briefing maps could create a common operating picture.

- The 2004 Indian Ocean earthquake and tsunami response
  taught us the value of a digital one-stop repository for
  geospatial data.

- The 2013 flu season taught us that additional insight could
  be derived from crowdsourced information and social
  media feeds.

Lessons learned from the pandemic

The lessons learned from the COVID-19 response have been considerable. Those insights are shaped by new technologies available
to collect data, the depth and breadth of economic data needed to
balance reopening and recovery phases, and statistical models that
guided key decisions. Crowdsourced information gave insight into
economic conditions such as the location of closed businesses and
daycare options for essential workers. Location-based human movement data provided a window into crowd surges and social distancing behaviors. There was an increasing need to identify testing and
vaccination centers, maintain their supplies, and determine their opti-
mal locations based on at-risk populations. The pandemic introduced
the terms "essential worker" and "essential business" and emphasized social distancing and protective face masks. Fresh partnerships
and innovative data providers emerged to support tracking and metrics associated with these novel concepts and challenges.

One of the hallmarks of the pandemic has been the need for speed. Its rapid spread required not the perfect plan but an immediate one. That meant actionable information, not just a flood of data. GIS allowed state and local governments to react quickly to the pandemic. Automating workflows tends to be the most common application need during an emergency. Automation can be as simple as launching applications to collect authoritative data on building conditions, hospital capacity, and bed availability; identifying the location and supply levels of resources; and assessing population risk and need. Applications such as these have been foundational to recent recovery efforts ranging from the eradication of Ebola in West Africa in 2016 and hepatitis A among homeless populations in San Diego County in 2018.

The efforts surrounding COVID-19 required new applications and related models to help keep the virus in check. For example, the operations dashboard became the most predominant tool used worldwide for disease monitoring and public communication. Along the way came applications to help the business community monitor workforce availability and supply chains. For instance, applications emerged for modeling indoor operations and space planning to help workers return safely to the office and for travelers to move inside airports and transit stations. Community contact tracing merged old data collection processes with GIS to provide quick, new insights.

As waves of the pandemic surged and receded, it became clear that every public health plan must expand to include these core competencies:

- Embrace broader cooperation
- Accommodate shifts in data needs and models
- Automate common workflows with maps and apps

Broader collaboration

Lessons learned:

- Reassess the list of stakeholders who must be included in decision-making.
- Acknowledge the repeatable patterns and workflows that peers use.
- Add economic recovery and reopening of communities to the preparedness plans.
- Examine how business and government decisions may impact people.

Shifts in data needs and models

Lessons learned:

- Include data related to essential workers, essential businesses, and at-risk populations.
- Monitor and model economic data such as business status and employment.
- Use sensor and crowdsourced data, such as human movement and business open rates, to augment existing data.

Automating common workflows with maps and apps

Lessons learned:

- Use mobile solutions to address inventory, capacity tracking, and all types of rapid data collection needs.
- Expand spatial thinking to the indoor environment.
- Consider workforce and supply chain management as important elements in any response.

- Create communication hubs to support decision-making and transparency.

Planning for the future

The health community advised disciplines such as parks and recreation, public works, urban planning, economic development, transportation, utilities, business, and even elections management as new collaborations formed to confront the pandemic. The result of this collaboration illustrates the holistic concept of "health in all policies." Going forward, we must cooperate at all levels, promote reciprocal sharing, automate processes, employ predictive modeling, embrace geospatial technologies, and include matters of equity in every decision. We will need all these capabilities and more to address the global crises of today—and tomorrow.

NEXT STEPS

The geographic approach to pandemics

THE USE OF GIS AND SPATIAL THINKING IS WELL established as a unifying way to bring together disparate disciplines and systems and improve collaboration and outcomes. Extending location-centric data can further interconnect our world.

Events such as the COVID-19 pandemic have illustrated the ability of health and human services departments to forge stronger relationships with GIS experts and become practitioners themselves. The response to the pandemic also underscored the connection between public health and economic health, another argument for heightened collaboration. Making these connections in the planning phases can help the transition to more effective response and recovery. There is much to do, but how do you get started?

This section suggests strategies to develop a strong geographic foundation for managing pandemics and just about any other kind of emergency. Let's begin with the data. Why is it important? Where can you find it? What datasets should you focus on? How can you identify data gaps and fill them? Data is the foundation for the information products and map applications you'll need. The examples in this section can help kickstart your spatial thinking about information products. You can use them and the other lessons of this book to help address your own organizational needs.

After establishing your needs for data and information products, you can execute your plan. It's best to seek information on best practices at every step. Staff may need to build additional skills to be proficient in this work, so this section also addresses opportunities to

...ild capacity. In many cases, the application or information product has already been built. For example, ArcGIS Solutions is designed to accelerate your productivity.

This section ends by discussing the value of hubs for housing data and applications and providing stakeholder and public communications. Pandemic response requires more than deploying a single GIS tool or map. Effective response requires workflows—end-to-end processes necessary to accomplish a goal. This section will present a sample workflow to underscore that need.

The importance of data

The importance of data during a health emergency extends far beyond government agencies. Different people and organizations have varied perspectives and goals. They often want access to authoritative data sources to do their own analysis, deploy resources, build and run models, and evaluate decisions. Esri, in partnership with corporate, academic, and not-for-profit organizations, as well as federal, state, and municipal governments, has taken the first step in providing standardized information that's easily accessible as public datasets. This work continues with resources available on the Esri COVID-19 GIS Hub, ArcGIS Living Atlas, and ArcGIS Hub.

The health community will continue to increase and adapt the data it needs to react effectively. The following list includes some of the common and now foundational datasets required for responding to a pandemic. In time, additional data requirements will likely emerge.

Common data requirements for public health preparedness

To scope out the crisis:

- Health care facilities (hospitals, urgent care, nursing homes, and so on)

- Other facilities (schools, day cares, shelters, public health departments, and so on)

- Transportation networks and infrastructure (roads, helicopter landing zones, public transit stations, railways, ports, airports, and so on)

- Boundaries (postal codes, counties, states, health districts, FEMA regions, hospital service areas, and so on)

- Homeland Infrastructure Foundation-Level Data (critical national and community infrastructure as defined by the US Department of Homeland Security)

To map the spread:

- Cases (frequencies, rates, and so on)

- Deaths (frequencies, rates, and so on)

- Recovered (frequencies, rates, and so on)

- Projecting and forecasting cases, deaths, and resource needs

- Tagged social media, Google searches or related surveys, hospital reported data, wastewater testing, and purchasing behaviors (for example, medication purchases) to support broad surveillance activities

- Social distancing behaviors understood through anonymized and aggregated cell phone data

To identify vulnerable communities:

- Demographics (race, ethnicity, age groups, income, and so on)

- Labor statistics (unemployment and employment)

- Homeless population (from point-in-time counts and Homeless Management Information Systems)

- Essential workers mapped by job classifications

- Concurrent disasters that may present potential congregation points or the inability to quarantine or social distance (floods, wildfires, hurricanes, heat waves, and so on)

- Social vulnerability (transportation access, health insurance coverage, poverty, disabilities, predominant language spoken, access to broadband, and so on)

- Comorbidities and health outcomes

- Population cohorts at risk (children, older adults, and so on)

- School locations

To allocate resources:

- Potential staging and triage areas during medical surge conditions

- Temporary or emergency shelters or quarantine and isolation locations (for example, schools and dormitories, community centers, religious centers, convention centers)

- Testing and vaccination sites, points of dispensing (PO... medical countermeasures

- Food distribution sites

- PPE, testing, and ventilator supply inventories

- Available beds per facility

- Intensive care unit beds per facility

To engage the community:

- Business impacts (closures, reduced hours and capacity, face-covering and vaccination requirements, and so on)

- Voting locations

- Policies per city or county boundary (for example, stay-at-home orders, emergency declarations, mandatory closings, face-covering rules, travel restrictions, quarantine areas)

- Longitudinal case trends

- Ongoing community health and needs assessments

- Changes in government services and hours

- School closures

y data gaps

ce you collect and organize your data, it's time to assess over-
al data readiness with a data drill. A data drill is a multiorganiza-
tion exercise used to gain insight into how a community collectively
thinks about, manages, shares, and uses data during an emergency.

Data drills are developed and conducted based on operational
challenges involving data and are a valuable tool for disaster preparedness. Data drills can be designed around a specific scenario relevant to your community to ensure you are planning for all data needs.

Example scenario: A disease outbreak has rapidly progressed
to widespread status in a community, and public health officials can
no longer hope to contain the outbreak through contact tracing and
quarantine. A series of community-level interventions must now be
evaluated and implemented to contain the outbreak. Health officials
must overlay outbreak data with other location-based information,
such as public gathering places, schools, health facilities and services,
and transportation centers.

Here are a few things to consider in your data drill. Once you
complete the data drill, develop a plan to collect or create data where
required based on these suggestions:

- Detail your organization-specific operational workflows and
  use cases based on the scenario.

- Identify the relevant decisions that are needed and which
  datasets, including metadata and data dictionaries, support
  those key decisions.

- Look next at your interagency workflows based on the
  scenario and do the same—identify the key decisions and
  data needs.

- For each data point, identify the responsible organization contacts, roles, and responsibilities.

- Identify whether any data-sharing agreements will be needed between partners, and start collecting and sharing the data identified in this drill.

Information products lay the foundation for crisis response

The circumstances of a public health crisis make it extremely difficult to slow down and think in detail about what you need to support response and recovery efforts. By this point, it is too late to take steps to be better prepared. Public health preparedness should be an iterative process, with the experience of each crisis informing preparations for the next. The goal is to always be ready, although we'll never be totally prepared for each and every situation. Data readiness helps us to be agile and equipped to react to changing needs as they arise.

Part of our advanced preparation requires taking the time to consider what information products and applications could help organizations with the challenges they are most likely to face. Time and communication are the factors that typically impede emergency response.

Drawing from past experiences, apps and information products that can collect data, analyze information for quick decision-making, and support briefings should be at the ready. Based on the specific need, they may range from individual reports, charts, graphs, and maps to interactive dashboards that integrate multiple elements into a common operating picture.

Useful information products can be anticipated and configured before a crisis. Some of those information products and apps will be unique to an organization and therefore built to suit a particular eed. In many cases, however, responders encounter common patterns. Esri has already demonstrated numerous workflows that can save time and resources.

The next list includes examples of the focuses for many locationcentric information products and applications that organizations worldwide have successfully used for improving health response. These focuses include emergency management, vector-borne disease surveillance and response, and more.

Emergency management

- **Preparedness:** Understand risk and evaluate resiliency, increase response capabilities when a disaster occurs, and increase awareness throughout a community.

- **Response:** Address the short-term impacts of an event, maintain situational awareness, conduct initial damage and health assessments, prioritize how resources are allocated based on local needs, and inform key stakeholders and the general public.

- **Recovery:** Assess the full impact or extent of an event and return the community to normal operating standards.

- **Mitigation:** Reduce or eliminate risks to people, lessen the actual or potential consequences of an event, and reduce the effects of unavoidable impacts.

Vector-borne disease surveillance and response

- **Combat vector-borne diseases:** Understand vector habitat preferences, monitor disease presence from vector traps and sentinel animals, track spread in human populations, and manage vector control activities.

- **Response:** Understand the impact of infection presence and spread and share authoritative information about the situation with communities.

- **Recovery:** Monitor key recovery metrics and trends that support decisions on when to move from stay-at-home policies to phased recovery efforts.

- **Hospitalization and PPE inventory:** Inventory hospital capacity and the availability of PPE at local hospitals and acute care centers. Predict surge events and plan medical countermeasures.

- **Supply chain management:** Understand the flow of goods (vaccine, antivirals, PPE, and so on) from manufacture to point of use and plan for potential adjustments and redistribution needs.

- **Health needs assessments:** Engage volunteers, businesses, community partners, and community health workers to help assess the health needs of vulnerable individuals throughout a community.

- **Testing, vaccination, and food distribution sites:** Identify at-risk populations and develop plans to site needed resources, whether for testing, vaccination, food, or other essentials.

- **Business reopening:** Guide the decision to open or close a business location, ensure employee safety when returning to indoor spaces, and manage buildings during shutdowns and reopenings.

- **Small business recovery:** Promote small businesses operating during a crisis and understand the impact of the crisis on small businesses in the community.

- **Business continuity:** Maintain business operations and share authoritative information with customers and stakeholders.

Follow best practices

Pandemic responders have used GIS to collect and share information about COVID-19 through dashboards, apps, and maps. These applications have provided public information to hundreds of millions—even billions—of people worldwide. For example, the *ArcGIS Blog* reported that the Johns Hopkins University dashboard received more than 1.5 million views an hour during the week of March 8, 2020, at certain times of the day. Overall, it's been viewed trillions of times.

To ensure that your maps and apps are ready to handle the increased load from the public and media during a crisis and that your GIS environment is ready for the next response, you can follow the scalability checklist in "Essential Configurations for Highly Scalable ArcGIS Online Web Applications (Viral Applications)" on the *ArcGIS Blog*.

Learn by doing

Hands-on learning will strengthen your understanding of GIS and how it can be used to improve pandemic planning and response. Esri's Learn ArcGIS website, a collection of free story-driven lessons that allow you to experience GIS as applied to real-life problems, includes these and other pandemic-related lessons:

- **Visualize global COVID-19 trends in ArcGIS Insights**[SM]**:** Create maps and charts to determine where COVID-19 cases are located and how cases are changing over time.

- **Analyze COVID-19 risk using ArcGIS Pro:** Create risk maps for transmission, susceptibility, resource scarcity, and risk profiles for targeting intervention areas.

- **Create a COVID-19 relative risk surface:** Learn how to use the spatial analysis capabilities in Insights to create a COVID-19 relative risk surface.

- **Track virus spread using Insights:** Use link analysis to trace contacts as a virus spreads through a community.

- **Evaluate COVID-19 financial vulnerability:** Determine which areas are the most vulnerable to financial shocks caused by COVID-19.

- **Facility mapping for COVID-19 response:** Learn how to implement ArcGIS Indoors™ for COVID-19 facility mapping response.

- **Use the CHIME application in Insights:** Run a script and use the results to analyze hospital capacity in your health care region.

You can find these and other lessons for crisis response at learn .arcgis.com.

Health Information System Modernization: A GIS Curriculum

Another skill-building opportunity is the Health Information System Modernization GIS Curriculum. This online learning site contains hands-on tutorials to enhance the geospatial capacity of health stakeholders. By promoting training and technical expertise in GIS technology through the connection of maps, apps, data and people, the curriculum equips health professionals to make more informed health decisions. From fundamental GIS concepts to analytics, field operations, and collaboration, learners will gain a breadth of experience using GIS with multiple ArcGIS software products.

Get there faster with GIS solution templates

Whether you're in the planning phases of your preparedness work or you're in the middle of responding, GIS solution templates can improve your efficiency. ArcGIS Solutions are focused maps and apps preconfigured for common workflows. They are designed to improve your operations, provide new insight, and enhance service delivery. The COVID-19 pandemic inspired the development of many new GIS solution templates to help you get there faster and with less effort.

As an example, you can use the ArcGIS Coronavirus Response to visualize and understand the various community and organizational impacts of the COVID-19 pandemic and share authoritative information with the community.

As the COVID-19 pandemic spread, health and human services agencies were tabulating cases and testing results to better understand the effect on the community. To prevent further spread, health orders were issued that severely impacted services delivered to many public gathering places, such as schools, government buildings, hospitals, restaurants, businesses, and so on.

The Coronavirus Response Solution helps government agenc educate the public about those impacts. The solution delivers a se of capabilities that include tracking COVID-19 cases and response activities, communicating the impact on public places (such as schools and government buildings), monitoring meal programs and their supplies, and sharing information with the public.

The Coronavirus Response Solution includes these templates:

- **Community Impact Dashboard:** An ArcGIS Dashboards app used by health and human services staff to monitor key coronavirus response metrics and share this information with the public.

- **Community Impact Mobile Dashboard:** A Dashboards app, optimized for mobile devices, used by health and human services staff to monitor key coronavirus response metrics and share this information with the public.

- **Coronavirus Case Dashboard:** A Dashboards app used by health and human services staff to visualize coronavirus cases in their community.

- **Coronavirus Case Mobile Dashboard:** A Dashboards app, optimized for mobile devices, used by health and human services staff to visualize coronavirus cases in their community.

- **Case Reporter:** A Survey123 form used by health and human services staff to collect and tabulate coronavirus cases in their community.

- **Public Place Manager:** A Crowdsource Manager app used by health and human services or emergency response staff to manage the status of public gathering places (for example, schools).

- **School Closings:** An ArcGIS Web AppBuilder app used by the public to obtain school closing information.

- **Medical Facilities Locator:** A Web AppBuilder app used by the public to locate the nearest hospital or health care clinic.

- **Community Closings:** A Web AppBuilder app used by the public to obtain information about gathering places (for example, government buildings and public places) in the community.

- **Meal Sites Manager:** A Crowdsource Manager app used by school district or emergency response staff to inventory meal pickup locations.

- **Meal Site Report:** A Survey123 form used by school district staff or volunteers to tabulate meals served at a site.

- **Meal Sites Locator:** A Web AppBuilder app used by the public to locate the nearest meal site pickup location.

- **Meal Sites Dashboard:** A Dashboards app used by school district or emergency response staff to monitor meal programs.

Create coronavirus-focused hub sites for your organization

ArcGIS Hub organizes people, data, and tools to accomplish initiatives and goals in a cloud platform. It's like a website, but it's easier to create and has more built-in functionality. During the pandemic, thousands of organizations used Hub to share information and resources about COVID-19 with their communities. Examples include the Missouri Coronavirus GIS Hub, State of Maryland; the City of Durham and Durham County, North Carolina; the Matanuska-Susitna Borough; and the Indonesian Kawal Covid-19 Hub.

The Coronavirus Response Hub template was created to help organizations share updates about local response efforts. This template includes a mobile-responsive and accessible website to help organizations quickly and responsibly disseminate clear and accurate information for the health and safety of their communities. Similarly, the Coronavirus Vaccine Outreach Hub was developed to help health organizations build vaccine awareness and confidence, track vaccine distribution metrics, and provide information about local vaccine providers.

Build your own GIS workflow—example with vaccine distribution

One of the greatest challenges faced in the pandemic has been the massive vaccine distribution effort to reach every corner of the world with life-saving vaccines. Next, you'll find the sample applications from Esri that were built to support the CDC's *COVID-19 Vaccination Program Interim Playbook for Jurisdiction Operations*. Whether you're taking on a similarly immense project or simply working through a step-by-step process to distribute goods or services to your local population, similar GIS methods apply.

1. Evaluate local population phases

This example uses real-world data to determine population phases in a sample region. When a resource is scarce, it is sometimes necessary to distribute it in stages. Create categories of risk and use population demographic data to understand where and how many people fall into each category.

2. Assess current distribution sites

Next, the current reach of vaccination sites will be determined. First, you'll map the planned early distribution sites, most likely hospitals, clinics, and pharmacies. You must also decide on a travel time accessibility parameter. This can be anything that makes sense for the area—perhaps a 30-minute drive time or a 15-minute walk time. Because you've already mapped the underlying population phases, you can run the vaccine coverage tool to evaluate geographic accessibility of the vaccine (blue area) by the population of interest.

3. Select additional sites to fill gaps

The previous step identified gaps in access to vaccine with the planned early distribution sites. To fill those gaps and better serve populations, it is important to brainstorm all the possible candidate locations for vaccine administration. Those locations might be parking lots that could house pop-up or drive-through vaccine clinics. They could be schools, convention centers, libraries, or blood banks—any place in a community that could logically and logistically manage vaccine administration. Once those locations are mapped, you can add elements of equity that go beyond the geographic accessibility parameter we've already considered. What are the factors that might pose a barrier to your community members' getting a vaccine? You might add age, race, occupation, vehicle ownership, language, disability status, or anything else that seems relevant. These equity elements will be combined and serve as a weighting factor in the final

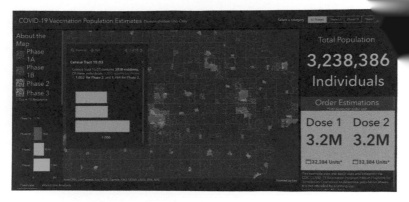

COVID-19 Vaccination Population Estimates dashboard.

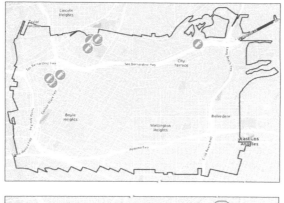

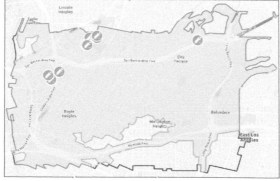

Vaccine accessibility maps showing existing vaccination locations (top) and population covered in a 30-minute drive time (bottom).

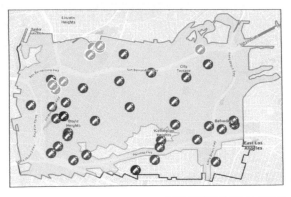

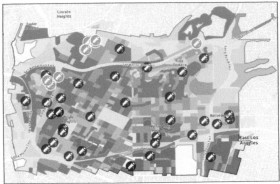

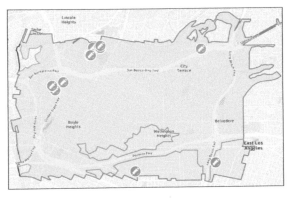

Three maps showing candidates for new vaccination locations (top, in gray), the combined equity elements for the region (center, where darker blue indicates higher vulnerability), and the best locations to fill the gaps (bottom, in green).

analysis. That final analysis selects the fewest of the candidate locations needed to close geographic gaps (in green) while favoring the sites with the highest vulnerability.

Ask for help

Everyone needs help at some point. In a pandemic, when just about every aspect of life is interrupted in some way, it's essential that we support one another. For additional support, many organizations have turned to the Esri Disaster Response Program (DRP). The DRP has provided GIS support to Esri users and the global community during disasters and crises of all types and scales for more than 25 years. The DRP can provide data, software, configurable applications, and technical support for emergency GIS operations.

Learn more

For additional resources and links to live examples and tutorials, visit the web page for this book:

go.esri.com/lfc-resources

CONCLUSION

PUBLIC HEALTH EMERGENCY PLANNING AND RESPONSE will always be an evolving field. The capabilities and processes developed in response to one crisis should build a stronger foundation for response to future events. The key is to consistently incorporate new tools and practices into existing workflows before the next crisis strikes.

Because of its scale and complexity, the COVID-19 pandemic has driven a range of innovations in health preparedness that we will draw on for years to come—and essentially move us to a new level of readiness.

This book has focused on one technology supporting that leap forward: GIS. This geospatial technology serves as the common denominator for any crisis because location data supports every phase of planning and response. GIS helps communities examine the extent of the crisis and predict the future course for allocating resources and monitoring processes and outcomes. GIS is the common language that enables public health organizations to coordinate efforts with other agencies and external stakeholders. In this book, we have shared several stories covering these use cases and more. Still, our learning goes deeper, so we conclude with a few more observations and nuanced lessons gleaned from applying GIS to the pandemic.

aring and collaboration

In this pandemic, we have witnessed the weaving together of multiple strands of information into a fabric of response that spans scales from global to local and crosses thousands of jurisdictions. We've seen unprecedented levels of collaboration, from the planet-spanning efforts of the World Health Organization to local hubs and dashboards hosted by innumerable municipal, county, and regional agencies. For years now, geospatial visionaries have touted the concepts of Web GIS; the spring of 2020 witnessed the realization of its potential. Modern technology can and should support our ability to come together with trust in times of need. The world is too complex for siloed expertise. Greater sharing and collaboration must continue as part of our future planning.

Networks and processing power

Those of us who lived through the rise of the computer age recall hulking, room-sized computers—less powerful than our smartphones—crashing beneath the weight of relatively simple tasks; poor, inaccessible, or nonexistent data; opaque, command-line software; and the tedium of digitization.

We still complain about the lack of data and its quality, and we still seek more powerful computers. But we've weathered bumpy transitions and now enjoy the benefits of decades of innovation. Data, processing power, and networked computing have enabled massive joint global efforts. If a hurdle remains to fully realize the potential of Web GIS, it's the inertia of institutions and our own failure to imagine and accomplish what these technological advances have made possible. We hope that the lessons in this book will support your imagination, ambitions, and experience as you put your own plans into action.

GIS and communication

GIS used to be almost entirely a back-office phenomenon, with highly trained professionals quietly laboring away using software and techniques only vaguely understood by the rest of us. The insights gained from their work benefited decision-makers within organizations but only occasionally reached larger audiences, and even then, only as abstruse, static reports and posters. Nowadays, GIS is as much about communication as it is about analysis. Web maps and apps have turned GIS workers into communicators. GIS has burst out of the back office to become an accessible, useful tool for organizations worldwide.

The GIS ethos

Literally thousands of hubs and dashboards have been published in response to COVID-19. Behind those efforts, and largely invisible to the public, is the work of legions of GIS professionals, gathering data, performing analyses, and assisting responders. Although their sacrifice pales in comparison with that of doctors, nurses, and others on the frontlines of the pandemic, their work is commendable in its own way.

GIS users often seem to have a certain kind of purpose about them. From health professions to every business that relies on location information—infrastructure, smart cities, public safety, conservation, education—these folks make their organizations more effective in serving a common good.

That same implicit ethos underpins and energizes ongoing efforts by geospatial professionals to help stop, or at least control, COVID-19. Looking at the countless maps, dashboards, hubs, and other pandemic-related resources, one can sense the passion of those who created them in the common cause to save lives and reduce suffering.

What this means for the future

The pandemic will likely be characterized as a period of social distancing and isolation, yet the crisis also underscored our interconnectedness and interdependence. For better or worse, we are a global community, and that means we must work toward understanding, planning, managing, and responding to global issues with as great a degree of collaboration as our diversity of viewpoints and backgrounds will allow.

It is human nature to fail to fully anticipate crises before they occur. We recognize that better planning would have dramatically reduced the impact of COVID-19. It is also in our nature to learn and grow and apply the lessons of one painful experience to reduce the impact of future threats. GIS holds the promise of being a central component of a global network that can sense threats, map their extent, and support solutions.

The public health preparedness community can make major inroads by embracing GIS data, models, communication and engagement hubs, and locationcentric applications. GIS technology is here to build on the past and propel pandemic planning and response into a better future.

CONTRIBUTORS

Matt Ball
Jim Baumann
Ken Blankinship
Allen Carroll
Chris Chiappinelli
Kymberli Fieux
Jhonatan Garrido Lecca
Kelly Gerrow-Wilcox
Gemma Goodale-Sussen
Diana Lavery
Jeremiah Lindemann
Keith Mann
John Nelson
Scott Oppmann
Monica Pratt
Mike Schoelen
Jeff Shaner
Jared Shoultz
Citabria Stevens
Christopher Thomas
Katie Thompson
Shannon Valdizon
Carla Wheeler

ABOUT ESRI PRESS

AT ESRI PRESS, OUR MISSION IS TO INFORM, INSPIRE, AND teach professionals, students, educators, and the public about GIS by developing print and digital publications. Our goal is to increase the adoption of ArcGIS and to support the vision and brand of Esri. We strive to be the leader in publishing great GIS books, and we are dedicated to improving the work and lives of our global community of users, authors, and colleagues.

Acquisitions

Stacy Krieg

Claudia Naber

Alycia Tornetta

Craig Carpenter

Jenefer Shute

Editorial

Carolyn Schatz

Mark Henry

David Oberman

Production

Monica McGregor

Victoria Roberts

Marketing

Sasha Gallardo

Beth Bauler

Contributors

Christian Harder

Matt Artz

Keith Mann

Business

Catherine Ortiz

Jon Carter

Jason Childs

For information on Esri Press books and resources, visit our website at esri.com/en-us/esri-press.